Extraesophageal Manifestations of GERD

Extraesophageal Manifestations of GERD

Edited by

Anthony J. DiMarino Jr, MD
William Rorer Professor of Medicine
Chief, Division of Gastroenterology and Hepatology
Thomas Jefferson University Hospital
Philadelphia, Pennsylvania

Sidney Cohen, MD
Professor of Medicine, Division of Gastroenterology and Hepatology
Thomas Jefferson University Hospital
Philadelphia, Pennsylvania

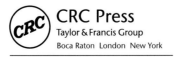

CRC Press
Taylor & Francis Group
Boca Raton London New York

CRC Press is an imprint of the
Taylor & Francis Group, an **informa** business

First published 2013 by SLACK Incorporated

Published 2024 by CRC Press
2385 NW Executive Center Drive, Suite 320, Boca Raton FL 33431

and by CRC Press
4 Park Square, Milton Park, Abingdon, Oxon, OX14 4RN

CRC Press is an imprint of Taylor & Francis Group, LLC

Library of Congress Cataloging-in-Publication Data

Extraesophageal manifestations of GERD / edited by Anthony J. DiMarino Jr, Sidney Cohen.
     p. ; cm.
  Extraesophageal manifestations of gastroesophageal reflux disease
  Includes bibliographical references and index.
  ISBN 978-1-61711-621-6 (alk. paper)
  I. DiMarino, Anthony J. II. Cohen, Sidney, 1939- III. Title: Extraesophageal manifestations of gastroesophageal reflux disease.
  [DNLM: 1. Gastroesophageal Reflux--physiopathology. 2. Gastroesophageal Reflux--complications. WI 250]

  616.3'24--dc23
                              2012046134

ISBN: 9781617116216 (pbk)
ISBN: 9781003524120 (ebk)

DOI: 10.1201/9781003524120

DEDICATION

We dedicate this book to our dear friend and mentor,
Dr. Edward Raffensperger,
July 9, 1914–October 2, 2009.

CONTENTS

Dedication v
Acknowledgments ix
About the Editors xi
Contributing Authors xiii
Introduction xvii

Chapter 1   Extraesophageal Reflux: Definition and Pathophysiology 1
               Vikneswaran Namasivayam, MBBS, MRCP and David A. Katzka, MD

Chapter 2   The Evaluation of Typical GERD 21
               John O. Clarke, MD and Donald O. Castell, MD

Chapter 3   Pulmonary Manifestations of GERD:
               Controversies and Consensus 35
               Lindsey B. Roenigk, MD and Susan M. Harding, MD

Chapter 4   Ear, Nose, and Throat Manifestations of GERD 51
               An Otolaryngologist's Perspective 51
               Joseph R. Spiegel, MD

               A Gastroenterologist's Perspective 57
               Lisa S. Cassani, MD and Michael F. Vaezi, MD, PhD, MSc

               Editorial: Point Counterpoint 72
               Anthony J. DiMarino Jr, MD and Sidney Cohen, MD

Chapter 5   Sleep Disturbance and Esophageal Reflux 75
               Christine Herdman, MD; Dina Halegoua-DeMarzio, MD;
               Sidney Cohen, MD; and Anthony J. DiMarino Jr, MD

Chapter 6   GERD and Oral Manifestations 85
               Mabi Singh, DMD, MS; Britta Magnuson, DMD;
               and Athena Papas, DMD, PhD

Chapter 7   Extraesophageal Manifestations in the Pediatric Population 97
               Joan S. Di Palma, MD; Sheeja K. Abraham, MD;
               and Rebecca O. Ramirez, MD, FAAP

Financial Disclosures 113
Index 115

Acknowledgments

The editors are very grateful for Dr. Papas and her contributions to Chapter 6. Also, to the expertise, professionalism, and patience of Carrie Kotlar, without whose persistence and support this book would not be possible.

ABOUT THE EDITORS

Anthony J. DiMarino Jr, MD attended the University of Pennsylvania and graduated from Hahnemann Medical College, where he was elected to the Alpha Omega Alpha Medical Honor Society. He completed his internal medicine residency and fellowship in gastroenterology at the Hospital of the University of Pennsylvania and served on its full-time faculty after training. From 1986 to 1996, Dr. DiMarino served as the Chief of Gastroenterology and Director of the Gastrointestinal Institute at Presbyterian/University of Pennsylvania Medical Center, as well as Clinical Professor of Medicine at the University of Pennsylvania. In April 1996, Dr. DiMarino was named the William Rorer Professor of Medicine and Chief of the Division of Gastroenterology and Hepatology at Thomas Jefferson University Hospital.

Dr. DiMarino is the author of more than 100 original papers, and as a lead author his papers have appeared in the *New England Journal of Medicine, Journal of Clinical Investigation, The American Journal of Physiology, Gastroenterology, The American Journal of Gastroenterology,* and *Gastrointestinal Endoscopy.*

Dr. DiMarino is editor-in-chief, along with Stanley Benjamin, MD, Chief of Gastroenterology at Georgetown University, of *Gastrointestinal Disease: An Endoscopic Approach,* an original 2-volume textbook, which is currently in its second edition, published by SLACK Incorporated.

Dr. DiMarino is considered a preeminent consultative gastroenterologist. In May 2007, Dr. DiMarino received the American Gastroenterological Association 2007 Mentors Research Scholar Award, which is given to individuals "who have made enormous contributions to gastroenterology through mentoring." Dr. DiMarino's research interests have primarily been in the areas of esophageal, gastric, and small intestinal motility; celiac disease; and the safety of gastrointestinal endoscopy. At the request of the Food and Drug Administration, he authored the "White Paper," which is currently still in use as the standard for reprocessing endoscopic gastrointestinal instruments to protect patient safety between patient procedures.

Sidney Cohen, MD is Professor of Medicine and Director of the Gastrointestinal Research Program at Thomas Jefferson University in Philadelphia, Pennsylvania (2001 to present). Previously, Dr. Cohen served as chairman of the Department of Medicine at Temple University School of Medicine in Philadelphia (1986 to 2000). His professional memberships include the American Federation for Clinical Research, the American Gastroenterological Association (AGA), and the American Physiological Society.

Dr. Cohen served as Chief of the Gastrointestinal Section at the University of Pennsylvania from 1972 to 1986. He was Chairman of the Department of Medicine, Vice President, and Distinguished University Professor at Temple University School of Medicine from 1986 to 2001. He was President of the AGA in 1991 and President of the Association of Professors of Medicine in 1996. He received the Julius Friedenwald Medal of the AGA in 2000.

Dr. Cohen is a graduate of Rutgers University in New Jersey. He received his medical degree from The State University of New York School of Medicine where he graduated magna cum laude. He trained in Boston during the 1960s where he was exposed to many of the great figures in gastroenterology who had a major impact on his career. He completed his internship and residency at Boston City Hospital in Boston, Massachusetts; his senior residency at The University Hospital in Boston; and his gastroenterology fellowship at Tufts University Medical School, New England Medical Center Hospital in Boston.

Dr. Cohen has authored and coauthored more than 400 original papers, abstracts, editorials, reviews, and book chapters on a wide range of digestive disease issues. His most recent publications include "Eosinophilic Esophagitis Presenting as Spontaneous Esophageal Rupture (Boerhaave's Syndrome)" in *Clinical Gastroenterology and Hepatology* and "Closure of a Nonhealing Gastrocutaneous Fistula Using an Endoscopic Clip" in *Southern Medical Journal*. His research focus is in the area of smooth muscle physiology and gastrointestinal motor function.

CONTRIBUTING AUTHORS

Sheeja K. Abraham, MD (Chapter 7)
Attending Physician
Pediatric Gastroenterology and Nutrition
Nemours Children's Clinic/Alfred I. DuPont Hospital for Children
Assistant Professor of Pediatrics
Thomas Jefferson University
College of Medicine
Philadelphia, Pennsylvania

Lisa S. Cassani, MD (Chapter 4)
Clinical Fellow
Division of Gastroenterology, Hepatology, and Nutrition
Vanderbilt University Medical Center
Nashville, Tennessee

Donald O. Castell, MD (Chapter 2)
Professor of Medicine and Director
Esophageal Disorders Program
Medical University of South Carolina
Charleston, South Carolina

John O. Clarke, MD (Chapter 2)
Clinical Director
Johns Hopkins Center for Neurogastroenterology
Assistant Professor of Medicine
Division of Gastroenterology and Hepatology
Johns Hopkins University
Baltimore, Maryland

Joan S. Di Palma, MD (Chapter 7)
Attending Physician
Gastroenterology and Nutrition
Nemours Children's Clinic/Alfred I. DuPont Hospital for Children
Clinical Associate Professor of Pediatrics
Thomas Jefferson University
College of Medicine
Philadelphia, Pennsylvania

Dina Halegoua-DeMarzio, MD (Chapter 5)
Post-Doctoral Fellow
Division of Gastroenterology and Hepatology
Department of Medicine
Thomas Jefferson University Hospital
Philadelphia, Pennsylvania

Susan M. Harding, MD (Chapter 3)
Professor of Medicine
Medical Director
UAB Sleep/Wake Disorders Center
Division of Pulmonary, Allergy and Critical Care Medicine
University of Alabama at Birmingham
Birmingham, Alabama

Christine Herdman, MD (Chapter 5)
Post-Doctoral Fellow
Division of Gastroenterology and Hepatology
Department of Medicine
Thomas Jefferson University Hospital
Philadelphia, Pennsylvania

David A. Katzka, MD (Chapter 1)
Mayo Clinic
Rochester, Minnesota

Britta Magnuson, DMD (Chapter 6)
Instructor
Department of Diagnosis and Health Promotion
Tufts University School of Dental Medicine
Boston, Massachusetts

Vikneswaran Namasivayam, MBBS, MRCP (Chapter 1)
Consultant
Gastroenterology and Hepatology
Singapore General Hospital
Adjunct Assistant Professor
Duke-NUS Graduate Medical School
Singapore

Athena Papas, DMD, PhD (Chapter 6)
Professor and Director
Oral Medicine Service
Department of Diagnosis and Health Promotion
Tufts University School of Dental Medicine
Boston, Massachusetts

Rebecca O. Ramirez, MD, FAAP (Chapter 7)
Attending Physician
Gastroenterology and Nutrition
Nemours Children's Clinic/Alfred I. DuPont Hospital for Children
Clinical Assistant Professor of Pediatrics
Thomas Jefferson University
College of Medicine
Philadelphia, Pennsylvania

Lindsey B. Roenigk, MD (Chapter 3)
West Georgia Lung and Sleep Medicine
Carrollton, Georgia

Mabi Singh, DMD, MS (Chapter 6)
Associate Professor
Oral Medicine Service
Director
Dry Mouth Clinic
Department of Diagnosis and Health Promotion
Tufts University School of Dental Medicine
Boston, Massachusetts

Joseph R. Spiegel, MD (Chapter 4)
Associate Professor of Otolaryngology—Head and Neck Surgery
Co-Director
Jefferson Voice and Swallowing Center
Thomas Jefferson University
Philadelphia, Pennsylvania

Michael F. Vaezi, MD, PhD, MSc (Chapter 4)
Clinical Director
Division of Gastroenterology, Hepatology, and Nutrition
Director
Center for Swallowing and Esophageal Disorders
Director
Clinical Research
Vanderbilt University Medical Center
Nashville, Tennessee

INTRODUCTION

In the past 30 years, gastroesophageal reflux disease (GERD) has become an important area of clinical medicine. The interest began with the introduction of histamine receptor antagonists and later with proton pump inhibitors (PPIs). The suppression of acid secretion focused clinical attention on acid secretion as the major culprit of GERD. The disorder, for the purpose of all clinical trials, was defined as a clinical condition manifested by the symptom of heartburn and the sequelae of peptic esophagitis, stricture, Barrett's esophagus, and esophageal adenocarcinoma. Clinical trials focused on symptom relief and the healing of peptic esophagitis.

These trials were highly successful and led to widespread use of these agents, especially PPIs. As new drugs were introduced, the marketing became extraordinary. Marked improvement in symptoms and the safety of PPIs further contributed to their success.

GERD became widely recognized and treated by physicians and then patients themselves with available nonprescription drugs.

Despite all PPI studies being focused on symptom relief and the healing of esophagitis, GERD has gradually become associated with other common but unexplained disorders. These conditions have been designated as the extraesophageal manifestations of GERD.

The extraesophageal disorders have become widely accepted in clinical practice. The evidence supporting the pathogenesis of these conditions will be discussed in 3 major categories: guilt by association, observed mechanistic studies, and therapeutic response to treatment.

Authors will cite the evidence to varying degrees and success. In the final analysis, response to PPI therapy has become the defining criteria. Unfortunately, this clinical approach becomes quite costly, especially in chronic conditions where treatment, not cure, is the major goal.

We chose the topic and the authors to give the reader recognition and balance in treating patients with common symptom-based disorders. Final resolution of some of the controversies inherent in these associations may require better diagnostic tools and perhaps better pharmacological therapies.

Extraesophageal Reflux
Definition and Pathophysiology

Vikneswaran Namasivayam, MBBS, MRCP and David A. Katzka, MD

INTRODUCTION AND DEFINITION

Gastroesophageal reflux disease (GERD) occurs when the reflux of gastric contents causes troublesome symptoms or complications.[1] The Montreal definition of GERD encompasses a wide spectrum of manifestations. These include esophageal syndromes, which are further categorized into those with esophageal injury and those defined by the presence of symptoms and extraesophageal syndromes (Table 1-1). This is an operational definition that acknowledges the disconnect between endoscopic evidence of esophageal injury (eg, esophagitis, strictures, metaplasia) and reflux symptoms that is often encountered in clinical practice, as well as the need to classify patients based on presentation, particularly in the primary care setting where access to further testing may be limited. The distinction between physiological and pathological reflux is ultimately arbitrary, though the latter tends to be nocturnal and longer lasting.

A wide spectrum of extraesophageal symptoms and conditions has been ascribed to GERD (Figure 1-1). This is largely on the basis of uncontrolled observational data and often reflects a coexistence of 2 common conditions as there is a 10% to 20% prevalence of reflux symptoms reported in population-based studies in the Western literature, depending on how loosely reflux is defined.[2] Data substantiating a causal relationship for many of the postulated associations are generally lacking, and antireflux treatment demonstrates inconsistent efficacy in the limited instances where data are available. The Montreal consensus recognizes reflux cough, reflux laryngitis, reflux asthma, and reflux dental erosions as having an established association with GERD. Unfortunately, it has been quite difficult to delineate which subset of patients with these symptoms has GERD as the root cause of their syndrome. It has also been challenging to determine the precise pathophysiology and therefore treatment of these potentially GERD-related syndromes, as the concept of direct reflux-induced injury is being challenged by that of reflex-potentiated damage to these extraesophageal structures.

DiMarino AJ Jr, Cohen S, eds.
Extraesophageal Manifestations of GERD (pp 1-19).

Table 1-1	Montreal Definition of GERD			
ESOPHAGEAL SYNDROMES		**EXTRAESOPHAGEAL SYNDROMES**		
Symptomatic syndromes	Symptoms with esophageal injury	Established association	Proposed association	
Typical reflux syndrome	Reflux esophagitis	Reflux cough	Sinusitis	
Reflux chest pain syndrome	Reflux stricture	Reflux laryngitis	Pulmonary fibrosis	
	Barrett's esophagus	Reflux asthma	Pharyngitis	
	Adenocarcinoma	Reflux dental erosions	Recurrent otitis media	

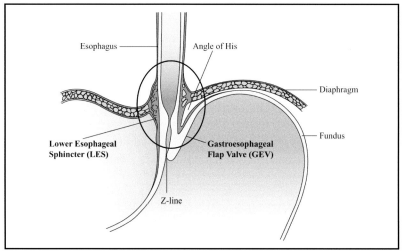

Figure 1-1. Schematic representation of 3 different mechanisms of gastro-esophageal reflux.

PATHOPHYSIOLOGY OF REFLUX

Gastroesophageal reflux is a physiologic phenomenon that typically occurs in the post-prandial setting.[3] Pathological reflux and its sequelae occur as a result of a dysfunction in the defense mechanisms protecting the esophagus from acid and factors promoting injury. Both symptoms and esophageal injury occur potentially as a result of proximal escape of gastric refluxate, impaired esophageal acid clearance, and increased susceptibility of the esophageal and extraesophageal mucosa to the refluxate.

Antireflux Barrier

The antireflux barrier is a functionally complex high-pressure zone that forms the main barrier against reflux. It prevents reflux of gastric contents during the interdeglutitive state, while allowing for the passage of air and fluids during swallowing and air with venting. It consists of the lower esophageal sphincter (LES), diaphragmatic crura, the intra-abdominal location of the LES, the phrenoesophageal ligaments, and the acute angle of His.

The LES is a tonically contracted smooth muscle at the distal esophagus composed of the major component of the antireflux barrier. The proximal portion of the LES is 2 cm above the squamocolumnar junction while the distal 2 cm is located intra-abdominally. Resting LES pressures, which range between 10 to 30 mm Hg relative to intragastric pressure, exceed the minimum pressure of 5 to 10 mm Hg required to prevent reflux, thus providing a reserve capacity.[4] The pressure is generated by the intrinsic tone of the sphincter as well as the excitatory cholinergic neuronal input.[5] The pressure exhibits diurnal variation and is highest at night and lowest in the postcibal state.[6] It may also vary with circulating peptides, hormones, drugs, and foods influencing the basal LES pressure. The LES is anchored by the phrenoesophageal ligament within the diaphragmatic hiatus.

The diaphragmatic crural fibers arise from the upper lumbar vertebrae and surround the LES at the level of the squamocolumnar junction. The crural diaphragm augments the resting LES pressure, especially during inspiration and abdominal straining. The crura fibers are independently controlled from the costal fibers of the diaphragm and are selectively inhibited during vomiting, esophageal distension, and transient LES relaxations (TLESR).[7,8] Impaired inspiratory augmentation of the gastroesophageal junction has been associated with GERD.[9]

The angle of His, on the greater curve aspect of the gastroesophageal junction, is created by the oblique entrance of the esophagus into the stomach, and it creates a flap valve effect that keeps the gastroesophageal junction competent.[10] Increased intra-abdominal pressure decreases the acute angle of His and compresses the infradiaphragmatic (intra-abdominal) portion of the esophagus, thus preventing strain-induced reflux.

Mechanisms of Reflux

Reflux occurs as a result of 3 mechanisms: TLESR, LES hypotension, and hiatal hernia (see Figure 1-1). These mechanisms may occur independently but all tend to coexist in more severe forms of gastroesophageal reflux.

TLESR (Figure 1-2) occur in the interdeglutitive period and are facilitated by both intrinsic LES and crural diaphragm relaxation.[11] Unlike swallow-induced LES relaxation, they are longer lasting (> 10 seconds) and not associated with peristalsis but instead are associated with distal esophageal shortening due to longitudinal muscle contraction.[12] TLESR is a vago-vagal reflex mediated by afferent fibers in the cardia in response to distension of the proximal stomach.[13] They are believed to be a physiological venting mechanism[14] and represent the main mechanism for gastroesophageal reflux. Of note, TLESR are not increased in patients with GERD compared to healthy subjects.[15] However, acid reflux as opposed to gas reflux is more likely to occur in GERD patients compared to normal subjects during a TLESR.[16] Some authors have hypothesized that this is due to an increased sphincter opening diameter during TLESR in patients with reflux when compared to normal controls.[17]

In contrast, reflux during a swallow-induced LES relaxation is uncommon as the LES relaxation is shorter in duration, associated with an esophageal peristaltic wave, and there is no inhibition of the crural diaphragm during swallowing. Reflux may occur during a swallow in the setting of a defective peristaltic wave or a hiatal hernia.[18,19]

Figure 1-2. Schematic representation of the neural pathway underlying the triggering and control of TLESR. Sensory signals from the receptors in the gastric cardia, pharynx, and esophageal body are integrated in brainstem nuclei, which, in turn, trigger motor responses in the LES, stomach, pharynx, and esophageal body and inhibition of the crural diaphragm. DVN indicates dorsomotornucleus of the vagus; LES, lower esophageal sphincter; n, nerve; NA, nucleus ambiguus; NTS, nucleus tractus solitarius. (Reprinted with permission from Mittal RK, Holloway RH, Penagini R, Blackshaw AL, Dent J. Transient lower esophageal sphincter relaxation. *Gastroenterology.* 1995;109:601-610.)

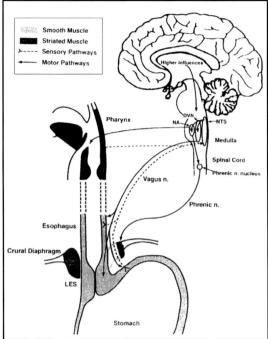

Reflux can occur in the setting of a hypotensive LES either as free reflux or strain-induced reflux. The latter occurs when the LES pressure is overcome by an abrupt increase in abdominal pressure. This usually occurs when the LES pressure is less than 10 mm Hg and in the setting of a hiatal hernia.[20-22] Free reflux refers to a drop in intraesophageal pH without a concomitant change in LES pressure or intragastric pressure. These are observed when the LES pressure is less than 5 mm Hg.

The presence of a sliding hiatal hernia is a risk factor associated with GERD. The barrier function of the gastroesophageal junction is compromised when the high-pressure zones created by the crural diaphragm and LES are separated in the setting of a hiatal hernia.[23] For the same degree of distension, the gastroesophageal junction may open wider in patients with hiatal hernia compared to those without.[17] This may partly account for the inability of the gastroesophageal junction to discriminate refluxed gastric juice from vented air in GERD patients, which results in proportionally more acid reflux with each TLESR in patients with GERD as compared to healthy volunteers. The presence of a hiatal hernia is also associated with more prolonged esophageal acid exposure due to poor clearance and a reduced threshold to TLESR. Furthermore, superimposed reflux may occur with deglutitive relaxation in the presence of hiatal hernia within which gastric acid may have accumulated.[19]

Several of the above refluxogenic mechanisms have been implicated in explaining the link between obesity and GERD. GERD is more prevalent in obese patients and obesity is also associated with GERD complications such as erosive esophagitis, Barrett's esophagus, and esophageal adenocarcinoma.[24,25] Central adiposity may be more important than body mass index in explaining the propensity for developing reflux.[26,27] Central adiposity may cause an increased intragastric pressure. Visceral fat is also more metabolically active and produces cytokines (eg, interleukin-6 and tumor necrosis factor-α), which may affect esophagogastric motor activity. LES pressure is lower in obese patients compared to controls, and a strong inverse relationship has been documented between body mass index and LES pressure.[28,29] Obese individuals also have increased TLESR that are also more likely

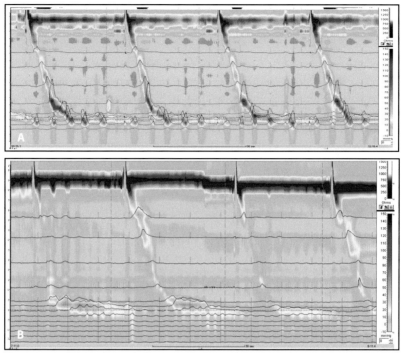

Figure 1-3. (A) High-resolution manometry demonstrating intact esophageal peristalsis. (B) High-resolution manometry demonstrating contraction drop out in ineffective esophageal peristalsis.

to be associated with acid reflux.[30] Obese patients have a high prevalence of hiatal hernia and, in turn, have a higher rate of esophagitis and pathological esophageal acid exposure.[31] Esophageal motor abnormalities are overrepresented in obese individuals, mainly non-specific esophageal motility disorders and nutcracker esophagus, but the majority of these patients are asymptomatic.[32]

Esophageal Acid Clearance

The clearance of acid following a reflux event limits the duration of contact between gastric content and esophageal epithelium. Acid clearance occurs initially with primary or secondary peristalsis that empties the refluxate into the stomach. Esophageal emptying may be impaired with failed peristalsis and hypotensive peristaltic contractions (< 30 mm Hg). Not surprisingly, peristaltic dysfunction is associated with an increasing severity of esophagitis.[33,34] Alternatively, esophageal clearance of acid may also be impaired by the presence of a hiatal hernia, which is associated with reflux of acid from the hernia during deglutitive relaxation.[19]

However, complete clearance of residual acid requires primary peristalsis (Figure 1-3) and its neutralization by swallowed salivary bicarbonate. As a result, nocturnal reflux is often considered far more injurious than daytime reflux because of the uncommon occurrence of swallowing during sleep. Esophageal defense may also be compromised in conditions that impair salivary production, such as with xerostomia, which is associated with prolonged esophageal acid exposure and esophagitis.[35]

Esophageal Injury

Gastric Refluxate

Esophageal injury in reflux is mediated by the synergistic combination of hydrochloric acid, bile, and pepsin. Animal studies have demonstrated that acid alone in very high concentrations (pH 1 to 1.3) or acid in combination with small amounts of pepsin may trigger esophageal mucosal damage.[36] In humans, the degree of mucosal injury correlates with the degree of acid exposure in healthy volunteers, patients with nonerosive reflux disease (NERD), esophagitis, and Barrett's esophagus demonstrating a graded increase in acid exposure.[37] Furthermore, the excellent efficacy of acid-suppressive medication in healing esophagitis and treating heartburn attests to the primacy of acid-mediating reflux disease.[38] However, basal acid output is not actually increased in patients with esophagitis compared to normal controls,[39] suggesting that gastric acid hypersecretion is not a factor in the pathogenesis of reflux. Furthermore, acid reflux symptoms often occur in the postprandial setting when intragastric pH is least acidic as a result of the buffering effect of food. This is accounted for by the presence of an acid pocket in the proximal cardia that escapes the buffering effect[40] and is of an adequate volume to acidify the esophagus during reflux. While this acid may potentially serve a physiological function of killing ingested pathogenic microbes during mealtimes, the acid pocket has been shown to be longer in patients with reflux compared to healthy controls and is entrapped above the diaphragm (especially in the setting of a hiatal hernia), which increases the risk of acid reflux in GERD patients during TLESR.[41]

In addition to gastric acid, in animal models, bile acid has also been implicated in reflux and has been shown to injure the esophageal mucosa with acid in a synergistic manner.[36] Bile acid persists in the gastric refluxate even with acid suppression. Duodenogastroesophageal reflux shows a graded increase across the spectrum of GERD.[37] Perfusion of bile salts at a nonacidic pH can trigger heartburn.[42] Bile salts act as detergents that damage lipid membranes resulting in the release of intracellular mediators such as histamine.[43]

Mucosal Defense

The mechanisms that protect the esophageal mucosa from injury upon exposure to acid are composed of pre-epithelial, epithelial, and postepithelial mechanisms. The Bernstein test, which entails continuous esophageal perfusion of hydrochloric acid, suggests that an intact tissue defense can withstand the effects of acid contact for 30 minutes without any symptoms in normal individuals.[44] The mucosa is lined by a bicarbonate-rich mucus layer secreted by submucous glands. The secretion of esophageal mucin is increased with esophageal acid and pepsin.[45] Beneath this layer lies the esophageal-stratified squamous epithelium. The stratum corneum, which is the uppermost layer, has tight junctions that provide a barrier against penetration by acid. The epithelium is supplied by a capillary network that contains acid buffers that wash away noxious agents. Within the intra-epithelial layer, acid buffering is provided by bicarbonate.

Esophageal injury occurs when the mucosal defense is breached by acid and pepsin. This may present with endoscopically evident mucosal injury (eg, erosive esophagitis, strictures, or Barrett's esophagus). Even in patients with NERD who have an endoscopically normal-appearing esophagus, injury (eg, dilated intercellular spaces) may be seen on microscopy (Figure 1-4).[46] This refers to the presence of prominent fluid-filled spaces between cells in the esophageal epithelium, which, when dilated, are associated with a paracellular "leak" allowing for acid to penetrate the epithelium. These spaces are best seen on transmission electron microscopy, though they also may be appreciated on light microscopy.[47] The presence of dilated intercellular spaces facilitates acid entry. Once the quantity of acid exceeds the buffering capacity of intercellular bicarconate, acid-sensitive nociceptors are stimulated,

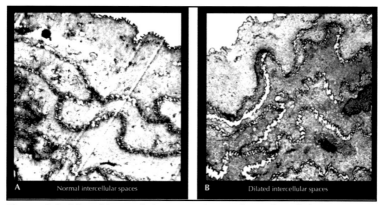

Figure 1-4. Dilated intercellular spaces in esophageal epithelium in GERD. (Reprinted with permission from Orlando LA, Orlando RC. Dilated intercellular spaces as a marker of GERD. *Curr Gastroenterol Rep.* 2009;11[3]:190-194.)

resulting in the perception of heartburn. In addition, the excess intercellular hydrogen ions result in intracellular acidity, which triggers a cascade of events ultimately resulting in cell edema and cell death. Cell death initiates tissue repair. When the rate of cell death exceeds reparative mechanisms, erosions develop resulting in erosive esophagitis.[48] The dilated intercellular spaces may reverse together with symptom resolution when proton pump inhibitor (PPI) therapy is instituted.[49]

Perception of Reflux

Growing evidence supports the concept that variations in visceral sensitivity to intra-esophageal stimuli is essential in causing symptoms of reflux. For example, patients with NERD are less likely to have an abnormal pH test than those with erosive esophagitis (45% versus 75%, $p < 0.05$) and have a lower number of reflux events despite having a similar or even increased rate of perceived acid reflux events.[50] The differential acid exposures, despite the similar clinical presentations of erosive esophagitis and NERD, suggest an increased symptom perception to similar or lesser amounts of esophageal acid exposure. This visceral hypersensitivity refers to the increased perception of gastrointestinal sensation in response to lower levels of stimulation. This may occur as a result of peripheral sensitization, central sensitization, and psychoneuroimmune interactions.[51]

Peripheral sensitization refers to the reduction in pain threshold to intraluminal stimulation at the site of acid exposure. For example, NERD patients have equivalent or increased sensitivity to acid infusion as well as increased sensitivity to weakly acidic reflux, compared to erosive esophagitis.[52-54] Mechanical sensitivity to balloon distension is increased in functional heartburn and acid hypersensitivity when compared to healthy controls.[55-57] Peripheral sensitization may potentially be mediated by the upregulation of acid-sensing receptors (eg, transient receptor potential channels [TRPV1]) in vagal and spinal afferents, as demonstrated in animal models of reflux.[58] TRPV1 proteins may be upregulated in esophageal mucosal specimens of patients with erosive esophagitis and NERD.[59,60] These channels that are located at the vagal and spinal afferents become more permeable in response to noxious stimuli (eg, acid or pepsin) with the release of inflammatory mediators like bradykinin, histamine, and prostaglandins.

Central sensitization refers to sensitization of spinal cord dorsal horn neurons after repetitive nociceptive signaling from the periphery that results in heightened response

Table 1-2	Extraesophageal Conditions Ascribed to GERD	
ESTABLISHED ASSOCIATION	**PROPOSED ASSOCIATION**	
Asthma	Laryngeal nodules	
Reflux cough	Laryngeal cancer	
Reflux laryngitis	Globus	
Reflux dental erosions	Pneumonitis/lung fibrosis	
Noncardiac chest pain	Sinusitis	
	Otitis media	

to both innocuous and noxious stimuli. This may also be associated with the recruitment of nociceptive receptors in adjacent spinal neurons that are remote from the site of peripheral sensitization.[51] NERD patients may experience hyperalgesia in the esophagus, stomach, and chest wall known as *spatiation*. Esophageal sensitization may also occur, as demonstrated by acid infusion in the distal esophagus, lowering the esophageal pain threshold in the proximal esophagus in patients with noncardiac chest pain.[61,62] Prior esophageal acid exposure may also cause symptom perception of acid exposures, which would be asymptomatic without prior acid exposure.[63]

Psychological stress and anxiety contribute to the generation of symptoms in GERD. The majority of individuals with heartburn reported, in a Gallup poll, a worsening of symptoms with stress.[64] Symptoms following acid suppression are also more common in patients with stress. Acute stress may increase sensitivity to esophageal acid exposure in GERD, while relaxation training decreases symptoms and sensitivity to acid.[65,66] Auditory stress and sleep deprivation worsen symptoms with acid infusion.[67,68] Stress may increase esophageal permeability and result in dilated intercellular spaces that expose the nerve endings to the refluxate.[69]

PATHOPHYSIOLOGY OF EXTRAESOPHAGEAL GERD: REFLUX AND REFLEX

The extraesophageal manifestations ascribed to reflux (Table 1-2) occur as a consequence of contact of the supraesophageal epithelium with aspirated refluxate or through vagal-mediated effects of the refluxate. *Aspiration* refers to the inhalation of oropharyngeal or gastric contents into the larynx and lower respiratory tract.[70] Aspiration of small amounts of oropharyngeal secretions during sleep is a physiological phenomenon that is compensated for by the normal host defense, including glottic closure and the cough reflex.[71] It is not known if this protective mechanism is altered in patients with reflux-related respiratory symptoms. Vagal-mediated reflexes have been implicated in the pathogenesis of various extraesophageal manifestations. This is a reflection of the common innervations of the esophagus, larynx, airways, and heart by the vagus nerve. The convergence of vagal afferents from the esophagus and the respiratory tract in the brainstem may provide an explanation for refluxate within the esophagus, stimulating extraesophageal manifestations such as cough. Both aspiration and vagal influences have been implicated to varying degrees in the various extraesophageal manifestations ascribed to GERD.[72]

Dental Erosions

Dental erosion refers to the chemical dissolution of enamel in the mouth caused by acid of nonbacterial origin. This occurs when the buffering capacity of the oral cavity is overcome by reduced salivary secretion or increased exposure to acid. The acid may be derived from extrinsic sources of acid, such as diet or medications (eg, vitamin C and iron), or gastric hydrochloric acid from reflux, rumination, or vomiting.[73,74] Dental erosion occurs when the inorganic hydroxyapatite crystals in the enamel are dissolved by reflux typically at a pH below 5.5.[75] Dental erosions are more common in GERD patients than the general population with a prevalence of 5% to 47.5%. Conversely, GERD is observed in 21% to 83% of patients with dental erosions depending on the method used to diagnose GERD.[76] The number and severity of erosions seem to correlate with the presence of reflux.[77,78] The progression of dental erosions may be retarded with PPI therapy,[79] lending credence to a plausible causal relationship between reflux and dental erosions.

Reflux-Induced Laryngitis

Reflux has been implicated as a cofactor contributing to laryngitis in addition to other irritants, such as tobacco, heavy voice usage, habitual throat-clearing, postnasal drip, and infection. The larynx represents the junction between the gastrointestinal and respiratory systems. The laryngeal mucosa exhibits greater susceptibility to reflux-induced injury from fewer episodes of reflux and more weakly acidic reflux, and increased susceptibility to pepsin, than the esophagus.[80,81] This may be driven by differences in the expression of mucin, carbonic anhydrase, and stress proteins by the larynx in response to reflux. The diminished carbonic anhydrase in laryngeal mucosa predisposes to a permissive acidic environment that possibly favors pepsin-mediated injury.[82-84]

Also, in contrast to the esophagus, the larynx also lacks effective mechanisms of clearing refluxed acid once it comes into contact with the larynx. Thus, it is not surprising that some investigators have demonstrated that minimally abnormal, or even physiologic, acid exposure may lead to laryngeal injury.

The assessment of the contribution of reflux in laryngitis has been hampered by limitations in the diagnostic modalities available to diagnose reflux. Laryngoscopic findings are nonspecific and often seen in asymptomatic healthy volunteers.[85] The use of pH testing is hampered by variability in testing methods and lack of agreement on normative values. The use of pH 4 as a cutoff at the proximal probe is undermined by swallowed saliva and airway secretions that may raise the pH.[86] Proximal pH monitoring has poor reproducibility.[87] The use of the LES as the reference for probe placement as opposed to the upper esophageal sphincter may result in inconsistent probe positioning due to varying esophageal lengths.[88] High placement of the proximal probe may also result in spurious pH drops from intermittent drying of the probe. Combined pH impedance monitoring suggests that a substantial majority of pharyngeal reflux events may be gaseous events associated with a minor drop in pH that may not be detected by conventional pH testing.[89]

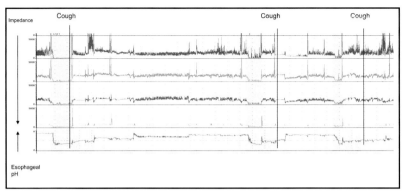

Figure 1-5. pH and impedance study demonstrating correlation between reflux episode and cough.

Chronic Cough

Reflux along with asthma and postnasal drip are the main causes of chronic cough, which is defined as cough lasting more than 8 weeks.[90] The diagnosis of the underlying etiology of chronic cough is often complicated by the absence of concomitant typical symptoms in an otherwise prevalent condition (ie, cough without heartburn in reflux or cough without wheezing in asthma). Emerging evidence, however, suggests that reflux is a cofactor rather than the sole cause of chronic cough, and it may sensitize to cough that results from multiple etiologies.

The cough reflex is triggered by inflammatory or mechanical irritants in the airways that stimulate various sensory nerve receptors. The afferent fibers from the receptors course through the vagus nerves and converge on the nucleus tractus solitarius (NTS). The NTS is connected to the central cough generator, which coordinates the efferent cough response. Cough may be influenced by the cerebral cortex facilitating volitional control of cough.[91]

Several lines of evidence favor reflex mechanisms or aspiration in explaining the relationship between cough and reflux. Acid infusion into the distal esophagus of patients with chronic cough increased cough frequency.[92] Topical administration of esophageal lidocaine blocked acid-induced cough, suggesting the presence of afferent receptors in the distal esophagus mediating the cough reflex. Furthermore, inhaled ipratropium bromide blocked acid-induced cough but not when directly infused into the esophagus, suggesting a role for vagal cholinergic pathways. Acid infusion into the distal esophagus increased cough reflex sensitivity in patients with GERD with cough, but not in GERD without cough.[93] Patients with a hypersensitive cough reflex demonstrated sensitivity to both capsaicin and citric acid inhalation.[93,94] Reflux-associated coughs correlate better with distal than proximal esophageal acid exposure (Figure 1-5), and bronchoscopy does not demonstrate evidence of microaspiration in GERD-related cough.[95] Patients demonstrating a temporal relation between reflux and cough had a more sensitive cough reflex than those without a temporal relation in the absence of any differences in esophageal acid exposure or erosive disease.[72] The esophageal-bronchial reflex is sensitized in patients with reflux cough, but it is unclear if the sensitization is driven by central or peripheral mechanisms. Infusion of acid and pepsin into the distal esophagi of rats stimulates afferent pathways that transmit signals to the brainstem, which could in turn activate efferent pathways.[96] The convergence of afferent input in the brainstem provides a plausible mechanism for various stimuli including reflux to elicit cough.

Cough has been associated with weakly acidic reflux (pH 4 to 5) in addition to acidic reflux, suggesting that the esophageal-bronchial reflex is activated by smaller amounts of acid relative to the amount of acid required to cause injury.[97] From a therapeutic point of view, this is problematic as it is pharmacologically difficult to maintain gastric pH greater than 5 consistently with PPIs. This might explain the relatively poor efficacy demonstrated by PPIs in the treatment of cough and the possible benefits of antireflux surgery albeit in uncontrolled studies.[98,99]

Cough may also precipitate reflux, thus setting up a self-perpetuating vicious cycle.[97] This would explain studies demonstrating an antitussive effect of antireflux therapy that persists far beyond the duration of antireflux therapy itself.[100] Coughing is a forced expiratory maneuver that involves a rapid increase in intra-abdominal and intrathoracic pressure, which may conceivably give rise to strain-induced reflux. However, a recent study using acoustic cough recording and combined impedance/pH monitoring showed that reflux rarely followed immediately after cough. The percentage of patients exhibiting a positive association for reflux following cough was reduced when the time window for symptom association was reduced from 2 minutes to 10 seconds. Furthermore, patients with a positive symptom association for cough preceding reflux did not demonstrate an increased likelihood of hiatal hernia.[72] This would argue against strain-induced reflux as a mechanism for cough-induced reflux. Whether coughing induces a vagally mediated increase in TLESR that provokes reflux is an intriguing possibility.

Microaspiration may also potentially cause cough by stimulation of laryngeal or trachea-bronchial cough receptors, but the evidence implicating direct microaspiration in reflux cough is limited. Patients with GERD and chronic cough have higher laryngitis scores and decreased upper esophageal sphincter pressures compared to GERD without cough.[101] However, a recent study did not document any difference in bronchoalveolar lavage pepsin concentrations between chronic cough patients and healthy volunteers.[102] The endoscopic assessment of chronic cough may be confounded by the traumatic effects of cough on bronchial histology.[103]

Asthma

The relationship between asthma and reflux is complex. Reflux is present in up to 80% of asthmatic patients, a higher prevalence than the general population.[104] This often occurs in the absence of any reflux symptoms.[105] The higher than expected prevalence of GERD in asthma forms the basis for speculating a causal link. Acid instillation into the esophagus induces bronchospasm in cats.[106] Esophageal acid perfusion increases airway reactivity without any effect on pulmonary function.[107] Microaspiration can cause airway constriction either directly or by causing chronic inflammatory changes that increase airway reactivity.

Conversely, bronchoconstriction in asthma may induce reflux, possibly by increasing TLESR.[108] Diaphragmatic descent in the setting of lung hyperinflation increases the pressure gradient between the abdomen and thorax and may compromise the barrier function of the LES by causing its herniation into the chest.[109]

Asthma medications (eg, beta agonists and methylxanthine bronchodilators) may have a permissive effect on reflux. Theophylline may increase gastric acid secretion and reduce LES pressures though the clinical significance is controversial.[110] Inhaled albuterol reduced LES tone and esophageal peristaltic amplitudes in healthy volunteers, but without any effect on TLESR.[111] A short course of oral steroids may increase proximal and distal esophageal acid exposure in asthma though the mechanism is unclear.[112]

The bidirectional interaction between asthma and reflux may potentially set up a self-perpetuating vicious cycle. However, a recent randomized control trial did not demonstrate any improvement in the control of asthma from acid suppression in asthmatics with asymptomatic reflux. Also, pH monitoring did not identify any subgroup of asthmatics that benefited from GERD treatment. Furthermore, acid suppression did not improve methacholine reactivity, suggesting that acid reflux is not a major mechanism of poorly controlled asthma.[113] Trials on asthmatics with symptomatic reflux have yielded conflicting results with no overall improvement in the control of asthma. These studies relied on patient-reported symptoms for defining GERD.[114,115] Thus, although there are several proposed and logical connections between asthma and GERD, a precise cause and effect relationship has yet to be defined in regards to mechanism and occurrence in patients with an overlap between these 2 diseases.

Pulmonary Fibrosis

Gastroesophageal reflux has been implicated in the pathogenesis of pulmonary fibrosis. Unlike cough and asthma, in which the vagal reflex is postulated to play a significant role, aspiration of refluxate is thought to be more important in pulmonary fibrosis. Pathologic reflux has been documented in 67% to 87% of patients with idiopathic lung fibrosis, with reflux symptoms correlating poorly with the presence of lung fibrosis.[116-118] Retrospective data suggest that fundoplication in patients awaiting lung transplantation resulted in stabilization of lung function, whereas control patients had deteriorating lung function.[119] There are insufficient data to support a causal relationship, however. Rodent models of chronic aspiration of gastric fluid showed histological changes that are distinct from those described in patients with lung fibrosis.[120,121] The reported prevalence of lung fibrosis is much lower than that of reflux[2,122] possibly because reflux is, at best, a surrogate marker of aspiration and patients may differ in their susceptibility to aspiration-related pulmonary injury. With the application of esophageal impedance monitoring to this subset of patients, a firmer relationship between reflux and pulmonary fibrosis may be defined.

Sleep and GERD

A bidirectional relationship has been postulated to exist between sleep and reflux (Figure 1-6). GERD may contribute to sleep fragmentation by awakening patients in the night or by causing multiple, short, amnestic arousals lasting less than 30 seconds.[123] Asymptomatic conscious awakening episodes without concomitant reflux symptoms may potentially be a manifestation of nocturnal reflux.[124] Conversely, sleep deprivation may enhance perception of intraesophageal acid, which lends itself to a potential vicious cycle.[68] Nocturnal reflux is associated with esophageal injury (eg, esophagitis, peptic strictures, Barrett's esophagus, and esophageal adenocarcinoma) as well as a higher prevalence of laryngeal and pulmonary manifestations.[125-127]

Sleep is characterized by alterations in esophageal function that have a permissive effect on reflux. Swallowing frequency is reduced during sleep, resulting in decreased primary peristalsis and, therefore, decreased esophageal acid clearance.[128] Decreased salivary production and decreased delivery to the distal esophagus during sleep retards neutralization of esophageal pH after acid reflux. Basal upper esophageal sphincter pressure diminishes during deep sleep, facilitating aspiration.[129] Gastric acid secretion is increased while gastric emptying is delayed at night.[130]

Reflux primarily occurs during stage II of sleep and rarely during the rapid eye movement period.[123] Maximal esophageal acid exposure occurs during the first few hours in the supine period, mainly during the recumbent-awake period rather than the recumbent-asleep period.[131,132]

GERD affects the quality of sleep via 2 potential mechanisms. Nocturnal heartburn may awaken patients from sleep, and reflux may also result in amnestic arousals. These usually occur during an acid reflux event.[133] Amnestic arousals, unlike heartburn, are

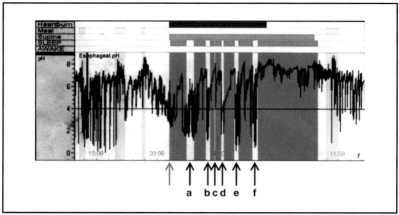

Figure 1-6. Blue shades indicate sleeping periods interspersed with 6 conscious awakenings that are associated with acid reflux events and heartburn symptoms (black arrows). The green arrow points to a short recumbent-awake period (green shade) that was also associated with acid reflux events. (A) 38 minutes. (B) 21 minutes. (C) 4 minutes. (D) 12 minutes. (E) 20 minutes. (F) 25 minutes. All conscious awakenings were associated with heartburn, resulting in a long, solid, red line. (Reprinted with permission from Poh CH, Allen L, Gasiorowska A, et al. Conscious awakenings are commonly associated with acid reflux events in patients with gastroesophageal reflux disease. *Clin Gastroenterol Hepatol.* 2010;8:851-857.)

not associated with reflux-attenuating behavior such as swallowing, rising up, or ingesting antacids, and this may potentially predispose the patient to the deleterious effects of reflux. The role of nonacid reflux in sleep disturbance is unclear.

Obstructive Sleep Apnea

Obstructive sleep apnea (OSA) is characterized by pharyngeal narrowing and upper airway obstruction during sleep, resulting in repeated episodes of oxygen desaturation and brief arousals.[134] OSA is a common condition estimated to affect 4% of adult males and 2% of adult females.[135] An association has been suggested between reflux and OSA by a high prevalence (80%) of abnormal esophageal acid exposure in patients with OSA.[136] The direction of the cause-effect relationship, if any, remains to be ascertained. Treatment with omeprazole reduced the frequency of apnea attacks in a small randomized trial involving patients with OSA and pathological reflux.[137] Conversely, treatment with continuous positive airway pressure reduced esophageal acid exposure in patients with both OSA and GERD.[138] Both conditions also share a common risk factor in obesity,[139,140] and particularly central distribution of adiposity, that may plausibly mediate any observed association.

Conclusion

An increasing number of conditions have been associated with GERD often on the basis of uncontrolled epidemiological studies. However, compelling evidence to implicate reflux in a causal relationship is generally lacking. Reflux is increasingly viewed as a cofactor in a multifactorial disease process rather than the sole etiologic agent in several conditions. Existing evidence invokes a varying combination of aspiration and vagal-mediated reflexes in explaining the link between reflux and the various diseases. Routine evaluation for

GERD as a factor in extraesophageal diseases is confounded by diagnostic paradigms that assume the esophagus as the site of organ injury and symptom genesis, reflux as a surrogate for aspiration, and acid as a surrogate marker for the noxiousness of the refluxate. These assumptions need to be revisited in defining the diagnostic threshold for peptic injury outside the esophagus.

REFERENCES

1. Vakil N, van Zanten SV, Kahrilas P, Dent J, Jones R. The Montreal definition and classification of gastroesophageal reflux disease: a global evidence-based consensus. *Am J Gastroenterol*. 2006;101(8):1900-1920; quiz 43.
2. Dent J, El-Serag HB, Wallander MA, Johansson S. Epidemiology of gastro-oesophageal reflux disease: a systematic review. *Gut*. 2005;54(5):710-717.
3. Demeester TR, Johnson LF, Joseph GJ, Toscano MS, Hall AW, Skinner DB. Patterns of gastroesophageal reflux in health and disease. *Ann Surg*. 1976;184(4):459-470.
4. Dodds WJ, Dent J, Hogan WJ, et al. Mechanisms of gastroesophageal reflux in patients with reflux esophagitis. *N Engl J Med*. 1982;307(25):1547-1552.
5. Dodds WJ, Dent J, Hogan WJ, Arndorfer RC. Effect of atropine on esophageal motor function in humans. *Am J Physiol*. 1981;240(4):G290-G296.
6. Dent J, Dodds WJ, Friedman RH, et al. Mechanism of gastroesophageal reflux in recumbent asymptomatic human subjects. *J Clin Invest*. 1980;65(2):256-267.
7. De Troyer A, Sampson M, Sigrist S, Macklem PT. Action of costal and crural parts of the diaphragm on the rib cage in dog. *J Appl Physiol*. 1982;53(1):30-39.
8. Altschuler SM, Boyle JT, Nixon TE, Pack AI, Cohen S. Simultaneous reflex inhibition of lower esophageal sphincter and crural diaphragm in cats. *Am J Physiol*. 1985;249(5 pt 1):G586-G591.
9. Pandolfino JE, Kim H, Ghosh SK, Clarke JO, Zhang Q, Kahrilas PJ. High-resolution manometry of the EGJ: an analysis of crural diaphragm function in GERD. *Am J Gastroenterol*. 2007;102(5):1056-1063.
10. Hill LD, Kozarek RA, Kraemer SJ, et al. The gastroesophageal flap valve: in vitro and in vivo observations. *Gastrointest Endosc*. 1996;44(5):541-547.
11. Holloway RH, Penagini R, Ireland AC. Criteria for objective definition of transient lower esophageal sphincter relaxation. *Am J Physiol*. 1995;268(1 pt 1):G128-G133.
12. Pandolfino JE, Zhang QG, Ghosh SK, Han A, Boniquit C, Kahrilas PJ. Transient lower esophageal sphincter relaxations and reflux: mechanistic analysis using concurrent fluoroscopy and high-resolution manometry. *Gastroenterology*. 2006;131(6):1725-1733.
13. Page AJ, Blackshaw LA. An in vitro study of the properties of vagal afferent fibres innervating the ferret oesophagus and stomach. *J Physiol*. 1998;512(pt 3):907-916.
14. Mittal RK, Holloway RH, Penagini R, Blackshaw LA, Dent J. Transient lower esophageal sphincter relaxation. *Gastroenterology*. 1995;109(2):601-610.
15. Sifrim D, Holloway R. Transient lower esophageal sphincter relaxations: how many or how harmful? *Am J Gastroenterol*. 2001;96(9):2529-2532.
16. Trudgill NJ, Riley SA. Transient lower esophageal sphincter relaxations are no more frequent in patients with gastroesophageal reflux disease than in asymptomatic volunteers. *Am J Gastroenterol*. 2001;96(9):2569-2574.
17. Pandolfino JE, Shi G, Trueworthy B, Kahrilas PJ. Esophagogastric junction opening during relaxation distinguishes nonhernia reflux patients, hernia patients, and normal subjects. *Gastroenterology*. 2003;125(4):1018-1024.
18. Mittal RK, McCallum RW. Characteristics of transient lower esophageal sphincter relaxation in humans. *Am J Physiol*. 1987;252(5 pt 1):G636-G641.
19. Mittal RK, Lange RC, McCallum RW. Identification and mechanism of delayed esophageal acid clearance in subjects with hiatal hernia. *Gastroenterology*. 1987;92(1):130-135.
20. Sloan S, Rademaker AW, Kahrilas PJ. Determinants of gastroesophageal junction incompetence: hiatal hernia, lower esophageal sphincter, or both? *Ann Intern Med*. 1992;117(12):977-982.
21. Dent J, Dodds WJ, Hogan WJ, Toouli J. Factors that influence induction of gastroesophageal reflux in normal human subjects. *Dig Dis Sci*. 1988;33(3):270-275.
22. van Herwaarden MA, Samsom M, Smout AJ. Excess gastroesophageal reflux in patients with hiatus hernia is caused by mechanisms other than transient LES relaxations. *Gastroenterology*. 2000;119(6):1439-1446.
23. Kahrilas PJ, Lin S, Chen J, Manka M. The effect of hiatus hernia on gastro-oesophageal junction pressure. *Gut*. 1999;44(4):476-482.

24. El-Serag HB, Graham DY, Satia JA, Rabeneck L. Obesity is an independent risk factor for GERD symptoms and erosive esophagitis. *Am J Gastroenterol.* 2005;100(6):1243-1250.

25. Veugelers PJ, Porter GA, Guernsey DL, Casson AG. Obesity and lifestyle risk factors for gastroesophageal reflux disease, Barrett esophagus and esophageal adenocarcinoma. *Dis Esophagus.* 2006;19(5):321-328.

26. El-Serag HB, Kvapil P, Hacken-Bitar J, Kramer JR. Abdominal obesity and the risk of Barrett's esophagus. *Am J Gastroenterol.* 2005;100(10):2151-2156.

27. El-Serag HB, Ergun GA, Pandolfino J, Fitzgerald S, Tran T, Kramer JR. Obesity increases oesophageal acid exposure. *Gut.* 2007;56(6):749-755.

28. Iovino P, Angrisani L, Tremolaterra F, et al. Abnormal esophageal acid exposure is common in morbidly obese patients and improves after a successful Lap-band system implantation. *Surg Endosc.* 2002;16(11):1631-1635.

29. Kouklakis G, Moschos J, Kountouras J, Mpoumponaris A, Molyvas E, Minopoulos G. Relationship between obesity and gastroesophageal reflux disease as recorded by 3-hour esophageal pH monitoring. *Rom J Gastroenterol.* 2005;14(2):117-121.

30. Wu JC, Mui LM, Cheung CM, Chan Y, Sung JJ. Obesity is associated with increased transient lower esophageal sphincter relaxation. *Gastroenterology.* 2007;132(3):883-889.

31. Suter M, Dorta G, Giusti V, Calmes JM. Gastro-esophageal reflux and esophageal motility disorders in morbidly obese patients. *Obes Surg.* 2004;14(7):959-966.

32. Jaffin BW, Knoepflmacher P, Greenstein R. High prevalence of asymptomatic esophageal motility disorders among morbidly obese patients. *Obes Surg.* 1999;9(4):390-395.

33. Kahrilas PJ, Dodds WJ, Hogan WJ. Effect of peristaltic dysfunction on esophageal volume clearance. *Gastroenterology.* 1988;94(1):73-80.

34. Kahrilas PJ, Dodds WJ, Hogan WJ, Kern M, Arndorfer RC, Reece A. Esophageal peristaltic dysfunction in peptic esophagitis. *Gastroenterology.* 1986;91(4):897-904.

35. Korsten MA, Rosman AS, Fishbein S, Shlein RD, Goldberg HE, Biener A. Chronic xerostomia increases esophageal acid exposure and is associated with esophageal injury. *Am J Med.* 1991;90(6):701-706.

36. Vaezi MF, Singh S, Richter JE. Role of acid and duodenogastric reflux in esophageal mucosal injury: a review of animal and human studies. *Gastroenterology.* 1995;108(6):1897-1907.

37. Vaezi MF, Richter JE. Role of acid and duodenogastroesophageal reflux in gastroesophageal reflux disease. *Gastroenterology.* 1996;111(5):1192-1199.

38. Bell NJ, Hunt RH. Role of gastric acid suppression in the treatment of gastro-oesophageal reflux disease. *Gut.* 1992;33(1):118-124.

39. Hirschowitz BI. A critical analysis, with appropriate controls, of gastric acid and pepsin secretion in clinical esophagitis. *Gastroenterology.* 1991;101(5):1149-1158.

40. Fletcher J, Wirz A, Young J, Vallance R, McColl KE. Unbuffered highly acidic gastric juice exists at the gastroesophageal junction after a meal. *Gastroenterology.* 2001;121(4):775-783.

41. Beaumont H, Bennink RJ, de Jong J, Boeckxstaens GE. The position of the acid pocket as a major risk factor for acidic reflux in healthy subjects and patients with GORD. *Gut.* 2010;59(4):441-451.

42. Siddiqui A, Rodriguez-Stanley S, Zubaidi S, Miner PB Jr. Esophageal visceral sensitivity to bile salts in patients with functional heartburn and in healthy control subjects. *Dig Dis Sci.* 2005;50(1):81-85.

43. Vaezi MF, Richter JE. Synergism of acid and duodenogastroesophageal reflux in complicated Barrett's esophagus. *Surgery.* 1995;117(6):699-704.

44. Bernstein LM, Baker LA. A clinical test for esophagitis. *Gastroenterology.* 1958;34(5):760-781.

45. Namiot Z, Sarosiek J, Rourk RM, Hetzel DP, McCallum RW. Human esophageal secretion: mucosal response to luminal acid and pepsin. *Gastroenterology.* 1994;106(4):973-981.

46. Tobey NA, Carson JL, Alkiek RA, Orlando RC. Dilated intercellular spaces: a morphological feature of acid reflux—damaged human esophageal epithelium. *Gastroenterology.* 1996;111(5):1200-1205.

47. Solcia E, Villani L, Luinetti O, et al. Altered intercellular glycoconjugates and dilated intercellular spaces of esophageal epithelium in reflux disease. *Virchows Arch.* 2000;436(3):207-216.

48. Orlando LA, Orlando RC. Dilated intercellular spaces as a marker of GERD. *Curr Gastroenterol Rep.* 2009;11(3):190-194.

49. Calabrese C, Bortolotti M, Fabbri A, et al. Reversibility of GERD ultrastructural alterations and relief of symptoms after omeprazole treatment. *Am J Gastroenterol.* 2005;100(3):537-542.

50. Martinez SD, Malagon IB, Garewal HS, Cui H, Fass R. Non-erosive reflux disease (NERD)—acid reflux and symptom patterns. *Aliment Pharmacol Ther.* 2003;17(4):537-545.

51. Knowles CH, Aziz Q. Visceral hypersensitivity in non-erosive reflux disease. *Gut.* 2008;57(5):674-683.

52. Miwa H, Minoo T, Hojo M, et al. Oesophageal hypersensitivity in Japanese patients with non-erosive gastro-oesophageal reflux diseases. *Aliment Pharmacol Ther.* 2004;(20 suppl 1):112-117.

53. Nagahara A, Miwa H, Minoo T, et al. Increased esophageal sensitivity to acid and saline in patients with nonerosive gastro-esophageal reflux disease. *J Clin Gastroenterol.* 2006;40(10):891-895.

54. Emerenziani S, Sifrim D, Habib FI, et al. Presence of gas in the refluxate enhances reflux perception in non-erosive patients with physiological acid exposure of the oesophagus. *Gut.* 2008;57(4):443-447.

55. Richter JE, Barish CF, Castell DO. Abnormal sensory perception in patients with esophageal chest pain. *Gastroenterology*. 1986;91(4):845-852.

56. Drewes AM, Pedersen J, Reddy H, et al. Central sensitization in patients with non-cardiac chest pain: a clinical experimental study. *Scand J Gastroenterol*. 2006;41(6):640-649.

57. Yang M, Li ZS, Xu XR, et al. Characterization of cortical potentials evoked by oesophageal balloon distention and acid perfusion in patients with functional heartburn. *Neurogastroenterol Motil*. 2006;18(4):292-299.

58. Banerjee B, Medda BK, Lazarova Z, Bansal N, Shaker R, Sengupta JN. Effect of reflux-induced inflammation on transient receptor potential vanilloid one (TRPV1) expression in primary sensory neurons innervating the oesophagus of rats. *Neurogastroenterol Motil*. 2007;19(8):681-691.

59. Matthews PJ, Aziz Q, Facer P, Davis JB, Thompson DG, Anand P. Increased capsaicin receptor TRPV1 nerve fibres in the inflamed human oesophagus. *Eur J Gastroenterol Hepatol*. 2004;16(9):897-902.

60. Bhat YM, Bielefeldt K. Capsaicin receptor (TRPV1) and non-erosive reflux disease. *Eur J Gastroenterol Hepatol*. 2006;18(3):263-270.

61. Sarkar S, Aziz Q, Woolf CJ, Hobson AR, Thompson DG. Contribution of central sensitisation to the development of non-cardiac chest pain. *Lancet*. 2000;356(9236):1154-1159.

62. Sarkar S, Thompson DG, Woolf CJ, Hobson AR, Millane T, Aziz Q. Patients with chest pain and occult gastroesophageal reflux demonstrate visceral pain hypersensitivity which may be partially responsive to acid suppression. *Am J Gastroenterol*. 2004;99(10):1998-2006.

63. Siddiqui MA, Johnston BT, Leite LP, Katzka DA, Castell DO. Sensitization of esophageal mucosa by prior acid infusion: effect of decreasing intervals between infusions. *Am J Gastroenterol*. 1996;91(9):1745-1748.

64. The Gallup Organization. *A Gallup survey on heartburn across America*. Princeton, NJ: Author; 1988.

65. Fass R, Malagon I, Naliboff B, et al. Effect of psychologically induced stress on symptom perception and autonomic nervous system response of patients (PTS) with erosive esophagitois (EE) and non-erosive reflux disease (NERD). *Gastroenterology*. 2000;118(4):A637.

66. McDonald-Haile J, Bradley LA, Bailey MA, Schan CA, Richter JE. Relaxation training reduces symptom reports and acid exposure in patients with gastroesophageal reflux disease. *Gastroenterology*. 1994;107(1):61-69.

67. Fass R, Naliboff BD, Fass SS, et al. The effect of auditory stress on perception of intraesophageal acid in patients with gastroesophageal reflux disease. *Gastroenterology*. 2008;134(3):696-705.

68. Schey R, Dickman R, Parthasarathy S, et al. Sleep deprivation is hyperalgesic in patients with gastroesophageal reflux disease. *Gastroenterology*. 2007;133(6):1787-1795.

69. Soderholm JD. Stress-related changes in oesophageal permeability: filling the gaps of GORD? *Gut*. 2007;56(9):1177-1180.

70. Marik PE. Aspiration pneumonitis and aspiration pneumonia. *N Engl J Med*. 2001;344(9):665-671.

71. Gleeson K, Eggli DF, Maxwell SL. Quantitative aspiration during sleep in normal subjects. *Chest*. 1997;111(5):1266-1272.

72. Smith JA, Decalmer S, Kelsall A, et al. Acoustic cough-reflux associations in chronic cough: potential triggers and mechanisms. *Gastroenterology*. 2010;139(3):754-762.

73. Lazarchik DA, Filler SJ. Effects of gastroesophageal reflux on the oral cavity. *Am J Med*. 1997;103(5A):107S-113S.

74. Mahoney EK, Kilpatrick NM. Dental erosion: part 1. Aetiology and prevalence of dental erosion. *N Z Dent J*. 2003;99(2):33-41.

75. Gudmundsson K, Kristleifsson G, Theodors A, Holbrook WP. Tooth erosion, gastroesophageal reflux, and salivary buffer capacity. *Oral Surg Oral Med Oral Pathol Oral Radiol Endod*. 1995;79(2):185-189.

76. Pace F, Pallotta S, Tonini M, Vakil N, Bianchi Porro G. Systematic review: gastro-oesophageal reflux disease and dental lesions. *Aliment Pharmacol Ther*. 2008;27(12):1179-1186.

77. Schroeder PL, Filler SJ, Ramirez B, Lazarchik DA, Vaezi MF, Richter JE. Dental erosion and acid reflux disease. *Ann Intern Med*. 1995;122(11):809-815.

78. Benages A, Munoz JV, Sanchiz V, Mora F, Minguez M. Dental erosion as extraoesophageal manifestation of gastro-oesophageal reflux. *Gut*. 2006;55(7):1050-1051.

79. Wilder-Smith CH, Wilder-Smith P, Kawakami-Wong H, Voronets J, Osann K, Lussi A. Quantification of dental erosions in patients with GERD using optical coherence tomography before and after double-blind, randomized treatment with esomeprazole or placebo. *Am J Gastroenterol*. 2009;104(11):2788-2795.

80. Koufman JA. The otolaryngologic manifestations of gastroesophageal reflux disease (GERD): a clinical investigation of 225 patients using ambulatory 24-hour pH monitoring and an experimental investigation of the role of acid and pepsin in the development of laryngeal injury. *Laryngoscope*. 1991;101(4 pt 2 suppl 53):1-78.

81. Sharma N, Agrawal A, Freeman J, Vela MF, Castell D. An analysis of persistent symptoms in acid-suppressed patients undergoing impedance-pH monitoring. *Clin Gastroenterol Hepatol*. 2008;6(5):521-524.

82. Samuels TL, Handler E, Syring ML, et al. Mucin gene expression in human laryngeal epithelia: effect of laryngopharyngeal reflux. *Ann Otol Rhinol Laryngol.* 2008;117(9):688-695.

83. Johnston N, Dettmar PW, Lively MO, et al. Effect of pepsin on laryngeal stress protein (Sep70, Sep53, and Hsp70) response: role in laryngopharyngeal reflux disease. *Ann Otol Rhinol Laryngol.* 2006;115(1):47-58.

84. Gill GA, Johnston N, Buda A, et al. Laryngeal epithelial defenses against laryngopharyngeal reflux: investigations of E-cadherin, carbonic anhydrase isoenzyme III, and pepsin. *Ann Otol Rhinol Laryngol.* 2005;114(12):913-921.

85. Milstein CF, Charbel S, Hicks DM, Abelson TI, Richter JE, Vaezi MF. Prevalence of laryngeal irritation signs associated with reflux in asymptomatic volunteers: impact of endoscopic technique (rigid vs. flexible laryngoscope). *Laryngoscope.* 2005;115(12):2256-2261.

86. Dobhan R, Castell DO. Normal and abnormal proximal esophageal acid exposure: results of ambulatory dual-probe pH monitoring. *Am J Gastroenterol.* 1993;88(1):25-29.

87. Vaezi MF, Schroeder PL, Richter JE. Reproducibility of proximal probe pH parameters in 24-hour ambulatory esophageal pH monitoring. *Am J Gastroenterol.* 1997;92(5):825-829.

88. McCollough M, Jabbar A, Cacchione R, Allen JW, Harrell S, Wo JM. Proximal sensor data from routine dual-sensor esophageal pH monitoring is often inaccurate. *Dig Dis Sci.* 2004;49(10):1607-1611.

89. Kawamura O, Aslam M, Rittmann T, Hofmann C, Shaker R. Physical and pH properties of gastroesophagopharyngeal refluxate: a 24-hour simultaneous ambulatory impedance and pH monitoring study. *Am J Gastroenterol.* 2004;99(6):1000-1010.

90. Irwin RS. Chronic cough due to gastroesophageal reflux disease: ACCP evidence-based clinical practice guidelines. *Chest.* 2006;129(1 suppl):80S-94S.

91. Chung KF, Pavord ID. Prevalence, pathogenesis, and causes of chronic cough. *Lancet.* 2008;371(9621):1364-1374.

92. Ing AJ, Ngu MC, Breslin AB. Pathogenesis of chronic persistent cough associated with gastroesophageal reflux. *Am J Respir Crit Care Med.* 1994;149(1):160-167.

93. Javorkova N, Varechova S, Pecova R, et al. Acidification of the oesophagus acutely increases the cough sensitivity in patients with gastro-oesophageal reflux and chronic cough. *Neurogastroenterol Motil.* 2008;20(2):119-124.

94. Benini L, Ferrari M, Sembenini C, et al. Cough threshold in reflux oesophagitis: influence of acid and of laryngeal and oesophageal damage. *Gut.* 2000;46(6):762-767.

95. Irwin RS, French CL, Curley FJ, Zawacki JK, Bennett FM. Chronic cough due to gastroesophageal reflux. Clinical, diagnostic, and pathogenetic aspects. *Chest.* 1993;104(5):1511-1517.

96. Suwanprathes P, Ngu M, Ing A, Hunt G, Seow F. c-Fos immunoreactivity in the brain after esophageal acid stimulation. *Am J Med.* 2003;115(suppl 3A):31S-38S.

97. Sifrim D, Dupont L, Blondeau K, Zhang X, Tack J, Janssens J. Weakly acidic reflux in patients with chronic unexplained cough during 24 hour pressure, pH, and impedance monitoring. *Gut.* 2005;54(4):449-454.

98. Chang AB, Lasserson TJ, Kiljander TO, Connor FL, Gaffney JT, Garske LA. Systematic review and meta-analysis of randomised controlled trials of gastro-oesophageal reflux interventions for chronic cough associated with gastro-oesophageal reflux. *BMJ.* 2006;332(7532):11-17.

99. Tutuian R, Mainie I, Agrawal A, Adams D, Castell DO. Nonacid reflux in patients with chronic cough on acid-suppressive therapy. *Chest.* 2006;130(2):386-391.

100. Ing AJ. Cough and gastro-oesophageal reflux disease. *Pulm Pharmacol Ther.* 2004;17(6):403-413.

101. Rolla G, Colagrande P, Magnano M, et al. Extrathoracic airway dysfunction in cough associated with gastroesophageal reflux. *J Allergy Clin Immunol.* 1998;102(2):204-209.

102. Decalmer S, Stovold R, Jones H, Pearson J, Ward C, Houghton L. Relationships between microaspiration, gastro-oesophageal reflux and cough in chronic cough subjects. *Thorax.* 2008;63(suppl VII):A22.

103. Irwin RS, Ownbey R, Cagle PT, Baker S, Fraire AE. Interpreting the histopathology of chronic cough: a prospective, controlled, comparative study. *Chest.* 2006;130(2):362-370.

104. Sontag SJ, O'Connell S, Khandelwal S, et al. Most asthmatics have gastroesophageal reflux with or without bronchodilator therapy. *Gastroenterology.* 1990;99(3):613-620.

105. Harding SM, Guzzo MR, Richter JE. The prevalence of gastroesophageal reflux in asthma patients without reflux symptoms. *Am J Respir Crit Care Med.* 2000;162(1):34-39.

106. Tuchman DN, Boyle JT, Pack AI, et al. Comparison of airway responses following tracheal or esophageal acidification in the cat. *Gastroenterology.* 1984;87(4):872-881.

107. Wu DN, Tanifuji Y, Kobayashi H, et al. Effects of esophageal acid perfusion on airway hyperresponsiveness in patients with bronchial asthma. *Chest.* 2000;118(6):1553-1556.

108. Zerbib F, Guisset O, Lamouliatte H, Quinton A, Galmiche JP, Tunon-De-Lara JM. Effects of bronchial obstruction on lower esophageal sphincter motility and gastroesophageal reflux in patients with asthma. *Am J Respir Crit Care Med.* 2002;166(9):1206-1211.

109. Choy D, Leung R. Gastro-oesophageal reflux disease and asthma. *Respirology*. 1997;2(3):163 168.

110. Harding SM, Richter JE. The role of gastroesophageal reflux in chronic cough and asthma. *Chest*. 1997;111(5):1389-1402.

111. Crowell MD, Zayat EN, Lacy BE, Schettler-Duncan A, Liu MC. The effects of an inhaled beta(2)-adrenergic agonist on lower esophageal function: a dose-response study. *Chest*. 2001;120(4):1184-1189.

112. Lazenby JP, Guzzo MR, Harding SM, Patterson PE, Johnson LF, Bradley LA. Oral corticosteroids increase esophageal acid contact times in patients with stable asthma. *Chest*. 2002;121(2):625-634.

113. Mastronarde JG, Anthonisen NR, Castro M, et al. Efficacy of esomeprazole for treatment of poorly controlled asthma. *N Engl J Med*. 2009;360(15):1487-1499.

114. Kiljander TO, Harding SM, Field SK, et al. Effects of esomeprazole 40 mg twice daily on asthma: a randomized placebo-controlled trial. *Am J Respir Crit Care Med*. 2006;173(10):1091-1097.

115. Littner MR, Leung FW, Ballard ED II, Huang B, Samra NK. Effects of 24 weeks of lansoprazole therapy on asthma symptoms, exacerbations, quality of life, and pulmonary function in adult asthmatic patients with acid reflux symptoms. *Chest*. 2005;128(3):1128-1135.

116. Salvioli B, Belmonte G, Stanghellini V, et al. Gastro-oesophageal reflux and interstitial lung disease. *Dig Liver Dis*. 2006;38(12):879-884.

117. Sweet MP, Patti MG, Leard LE, et al. Gastroesophageal reflux in patients with idiopathic pulmonary fibrosis referred for lung transplantation. *J Thorac Cardiovasc Surg*. 2007;133(4):1078-1084.

118. Raghu G, Freudenberger TD, Yang S, et al. High prevalence of abnormal acid gastro-oesophageal reflux in idiopathic pulmonary fibrosis. *Eur Respir J*. 2006;27(1):136-142.

119. Linden PA, Gilbert RJ, Yeap BY, et al. Laparoscopic fundoplication in patients with end-stage lung disease awaiting transplantation. *J Thorac Cardiovasc Surg*. 2006;131(2):438-446.

120. Appel JZ III, Lee SM, Hartwig MG, et al. Characterization of the innate immune response to chronic aspiration in a novel rodent model. *Respir Res*. 2007;8:87.

121. Katzenstein AL, Myers JL. Idiopathic pulmonary fibrosis: clinical relevance of pathologic classification. *Am J Respir Crit Care Med*. 1998;157(4 pt 1):1301-1315.

122. Raghu G, Weycker D, Edelsberg J, Bradford WZ, Oster G. Incidence and prevalence of idiopathic pulmonary fibrosis. *Am J Respir Crit Care Med*. 2006;174(7):810-816.

123. Dickman R, Green C, Fass SS, et al. Relationships between sleep quality and pH monitoring findings in persons with gastroesophageal reflux disease. *J Clin Sleep Med*. 2007;3(5):505-513.

124. Poh CH, Allen L, Gasiorowska A, et al. Conscious awakenings are commonly associated with acid reflux events in patients with gastroesophageal reflux disease. *Clin Gastroenterol Hepatol*. 2010;8(10):851-857.

125. Chen CL, Robert JJ, Orr WC. Sleep symptoms and gastroesophageal reflux. *J Clin Gastroenterol*. 2008;42(1):13-17.

126. Lagergren J, Bergstrom R, Lindgren A, Nyren O. Symptomatic gastroesophageal reflux as a risk factor for esophageal adenocarcinoma. *N Engl J Med*. 1999;340(11):825-831.

127. Fass R. The relationship between gastroesophageal reflux disease and sleep. *Curr Gastroenterol Rep*. 2009;11(3):202-208.

128. Orr WC, Johnson LF. Responses to different levels of esophageal acidification during waking and sleep. *Dig Dis Sci*. 1998;43(2):241-245.

129. Bajaj JS, Bajaj S, Dua KS, et al. Influence of sleep stages on esophago-upper esophageal sphincter contractile reflex and secondary esophageal peristalsis. *Gastroenterology*. 2006;130(1):17-25.

130. Pasricha PJ. Effect of sleep on gastroesophageal physiology and airway protective mechanisms. *Am J Med*. 2003;115(suppl 3A):114S-118S.

131. Dickman R, Parthasarathy S, Malagon IB, et al. Comparisons of the distribution of oesophageal acid exposure throughout the sleep period among the different gastro-oesophageal reflux disease groups. *Aliment Pharmacol Ther*. 2007;26(1):41-48.

132. Allen L, Poh CH, Gasiorowska A, et al. Increased oesophageal acid exposure at the beginning of the recumbent period is primarily a recumbent-awake phenomenon. *Aliment Pharmacol Ther*. 2010;32(6):787-794.

133. Dickman R, Shapiro M, Malagon IB, Powers J, Fass R. Assessment of 24-h oesophageal pH monitoring should be divided to awake and asleep rather than upright and supine time periods. *Neurogastroenterol Motil*. 2007;19(9):709-715.

134. Orr WC, Heading R, Johnson LF, Kryger M. Review article: sleep and its relationship to gastro-oesophageal reflux. *Aliment Pharmacol Ther*. 2004;20(suppl 9):39-46.

135. Young T, Palta M, Dempsey J, Skatrud J, Weber S, Badr S. The occurrence of sleep-disordered breathing among middle-aged adults. *N Engl J Med*. 1993;328(17):1230-1235.

136. Graf KI, Karaus M, Heinemann S, Korber S, Dorow P, Hampel KE. Gastroesophageal reflux in patients with sleep apnea syndrome. *Z Gastroenterol*. 1995;33(12):689-693.

137. Bortolotti M, Gentilini L, Morselli C, Giovannini M. Obstructive sleep apnoea is improved by a prolonged treatment of gastrooesophageal reflux with omeprazole. *Dig Liver Dis*. 2006;38(2):78-81.

138. Tawk M, Goodrich S, Kinasewitz G, Orr W. The effect of 1 week of continuous positive airway pressure treatment in obstructive sleep apnea patients with concomitant gastroesophageal reflux. *Chest.* 2006;130(4):1003-1008.

139. Jacobson BC, Somers SC, Fuchs CS, Kelly CP, Camargo CA Jr. Body-mass index and symptoms of gastroesophageal reflux in women. *N Engl J Med.* 2006;354(22):2340-2348.

140. Morse CA, Quan SF, Mays MZ, Green C, Stephen G, Fass R. Is there a relationship between obstructive sleep apnea and gastroesophageal reflux disease? *Clin Gastroenterol Hepatol.* 2004;2(9):761-768.

The Evaluation of Typical GERD

John O. Clarke, MD and Donald O. Castell, MD

Gastroesophageal reflux disease (GERD) is the most common gastrointestinal indication for outpatient physician visits in the United States today,[1] and it is estimated that nearly 20% of the population experiences symptoms on at least a weekly basis.[2,3] Given the spectrum of symptoms and the massive number of people affected, it is impossible and unnecessary to institute a formal diagnostic evaluation in all symptomatic individuals; however, for some patients it is a necessity.

As per the American Gastroenterological Association, GERD is defined as (1) a symptom complex attributable to gastroesophageal reflux and of sufficient severity to compromise quality of life, or (2) endoscopic findings of erosive esophagitis, stricture, or Barrett's metaplasia.[4] If symptoms are typical, the patient responds to therapy, and no alarm signs are present, then further work-up is not warranted; however, if this is not the case, then work-up is warranted to prevent misdiagnosis, evaluate for potential complications of reflux disease, and evaluate treatment failures.

When diagnostic tests are employed, it is important to answer 2 questions: (1) Does the patient have abnormal baseline gastroesophageal reflux? (2) Is ongoing reflux the etiology of the patient's continued symptoms? Over the past decade, new technology has changed the diagnostic approach to refractory reflux, and wireless pH testing and intraluminal impedance monitoring have both become widely available. With the arrival of these techniques, there has been extensive research into their limitations and clinical utility. This flurry of activity and interest has led to new societal recommendations from the American College of Gastroenterology,[5,6] American Gastroenterological Association,[7] and American Society for Gastrointestinal Endoscopy.[8] This chapter highlights the different techniques available for reflux diagnosis and their relative pros and cons.

DiMarino AJ Jr, Cohen S, eds.
Extraesophageal Manifestations of GERD (pp 21-32).
© 2013 Taylor & Francis Group.

ENDOSCOPY

Endoscopy allows for direct visualization of the esophageal mucosa and is the only reliable method to exclude Barrett's esophagus or reflux esophagitis. In addition, endoscopy has the potential to reveal an alternate diagnosis, such as gastric or esophageal malignancy, peptic ulcer disease, eosinophilic esophagitis, or other infectious or caustic esophagitides. Of this group, eosinophilic esophagitis is particularly worth noting as multiple studies have shown it to be increasingly diagnosed in pediatric and adult populations. Clinically, in selected patients, it can be challenging to separate from reflux based on symptoms alone.[9-12] For these reasons, most authorities recommend endoscopy as the initial diagnostic study of choice for patients with gastroesophageal reflux in need of further diagnostic evaluation.[4,13,14] The American Society for Gastrointestinal Endoscopy has even gone so far as to publish a societal guideline with the following listed indications for endoscopy in patients with GERD: GERD symptoms that are persistent or progressive despite appropriate medical therapy; dysphagia or odynophagia; involuntary weight loss greater than 5%; evidence of gastrointestinal bleeding or anemia; finding of a mass, stricture, or ulcer on imaging studies; evaluation of patients with suspected extraesophageal manifestations of GERD; screening for Barrett's esophagus in selected patients (as clinically indicated); persistent vomiting; and evaluation of patients with recurrent symptoms after endoscopic or surgical antireflux procedures.[14]

When endoscopy is performed, the presence of typical findings of reflux esophagitis is diagnostic of GERD with a specificity of at least 90%.[15,16] However, the sensitivity of endoscopy for the detection of GERD is significantly lower, and it is well established that at least 50% of patients undergoing endoscopic evaluation for GERD symptoms in the primary care setting will have a normal examination.[3,17] This sensitivity drops significantly further in tertiary referral centers and when endoscopic evaluation is performed in the context of acid-suppressive medications, presumably due to the widespread use and excellent healing capabilities of proton pump inhibitor (PPI) therapy.[18,19] In addition, it is worth noting that GERD symptoms do not correlate with the degree of underlying mucosal damage, and the presence of a normal endoscopy does not exclude abnormal gastroesophageal reflux.

When performing an upper endoscopy for a patient with suspected or refractory GERD, it is important to describe the extent of injury either through detailed description or a validated endoscopic classification system, several of which exist for grading the endoscopic severity of reflux esophagitis. While these systems were initially developed for research purposes, they are useful in clinical practice as they provide a common language to describe severity of reflux injury. Presently, the 2 most commonly used classification systems are the Los Angeles classification (Table 2-1) and the Savary-Miller classification (Table 2-2).[14] The Los Angeles classification has been shown to have reliable intraobserver and interobserver agreement.[20] In addition, if the patient complains of dysphagia or suspicion exists for eosinophilic esophagitis, then it is essential to take endoscopic biopsies as up to 50% of eosinophilic esophagitis cases may have a normal endoscopic appearance and the diagnosis can only be secured with biopsy acquisition.[21,22]

AMBULATORY pH MONITORING

When symptoms are refractory to medical therapy or the diagnosis remains in question after empiric therapy and endoscopy, ambulatory pH testing has traditionally been employed to assess esophageal acid exposure and symptom correlation. Catheter-based

Table 2-1	The Modified Los Angeles Classification of Reflux Esophagitis	
GRADE	**DESCRIPTION**	
A	≥ 1 mucosal break no longer than 5 mm that does not extend between the tops of 2 mucosal folds	
B	≥ 1 mucosal break longer than 5 mm that does not extend between the tops of 2 mucosal folds	
C	≥ 1 mucosal break that is continuous between the tops of ≥ 2 mucosal folds but that involves < 75% of the circumference	
D	≥ 1 mucosal break that involves ≥ 75% of the esophageal circumference	

Adapted from Lichtenstein DR, Cash BD, Davila R, et al. Role of endoscopy in the management of GERD. *Gastrointest Endosc*. 2007;66:219-224.

Table 2-2	The Modified Savary-Miller Classification of Reflux Esophagitis	
GRADE	**DESCRIPTION**	
I	Single or isolated erosive lesion, affecting only one longitudinal fold	
II	Multiple erosive lesions (noncircumferential) affecting more than one longitudinal fold, with or without confluence	
III	Circumferential erosive lesions	
IV	Chronic lesions including ulcers, strictures, and/or short esophagus (alone or accompanied by other findings of grades I to III)	
V	Columnar epithelium in continuity with the Z-line (alone or associated with other findings of grades I to IV)	

Adapted from Lichtenstein DR, Cash BD, Davila R, et al. Role of endoscopy in the management of GERD. *Gastrointest Endosc*. 2007;66:219-224.

esophageal pH recording has been in use for more than 3 decades and has a long clinical tradition and extensive research publications to support its use. However, over the past decade, the emergence of wireless pH testing and intraluminal impedance monitoring has lessened the role of catheter-based esophageal testing evaluating pH alone. While catheter-based pH testing can still be employed to answer finite clinical questions, wireless pH testing and intraluminal impedance monitoring both offer greater sensitivity and have largely replaced catheter-based pH-only testing in most academic motility referral centers.

Wireless pH monitoring represents an important recent advance in pH testing. The concept is that an antimony electrode is incorporated into a wireless capsule that transits pH data telemetrically via radiofrequency to an external receiver. Data regarding pH are sampled every 6 seconds at one fixed point, and this information can be recorded for 48 hours without the need for a transnasal catheter. In addition, several studies have evaluated the potential role for extended pH monitoring with prolongation of the recording time to 96 hours.[23-27] This device can be placed transorally or transnasally, either with endoscopy or without; however, in practice it is usually passed transorally with endoscopy due to the size of the device and deployment catheter.

Wireless pH testing has advantages and disadvantages, and it is important to discuss each in turn. One clear advantage of the wireless system is that it is less conspicuous than a catheter-based system and makes it easier for patients to continue normal activities after placement (eg, work, exercise, and social events). Several studies have shown that patients who undergo placement of a catheter-based pH system change their activity thereafter in ways that could potentially decrease reflux[28,29]; however, that appears to be less of an issue with the wireless pH probe,[30-32] perhaps explaining the higher normative esophageal acid exposure values seen with the wireless pH probe (5.3%) as opposed to the catheter-based pH systems (4.1%).[33] In addition to being less conspicuous, the wireless pH probe also appears to be better tolerated than the catheter-based counterpart, with at least 2 studies showing clear patient preference for the wireless system.[31,34]

A second potential benefit of the wireless pH system is that it can be fixed in place and clipped to a specific point in the esophagus and, thus, may not be as sensitive to deglutitive shortening as a catheter-based system that is secured only at the nostril. As normative data are based on distance of the recording device from the lower esophageal sphincter, it is important that the pH probe position be standardized, as even small shifts in distance could affect test results. The accuracy of the wireless pH probe placement was assessed by Pandolfino and colleagues. In their study, patients underwent simultaneous wireless pH and catheter-based pH studies and also had endoclips placed endoscopically at the squamocolumnar junction. Fluoroscopy was then employed to measure the distance between the pH electrode and squamocolumnar junction. Using this technique, placement variability appeared to be less with the wireless system than with traditional pH catheter deployment.[35]

A third benefit of the wireless pH system is logistics. Because the device is placed based on endoscopic landmarks, it can be done without a baseline manometry, as opposed to catheter-based systems, which require a manometry to obtain accurate landmarks for catheter placement. The physical space employed by the equipment is relatively small and easily incorporated in an endoscopy unit. Interpretation is also relatively straightforward. Given these features, wireless pH testing represents a relatively easy addition to a gastroenterology practice that may not have the resources or expertise to develop a motility lab with manometry and other more complex equipment and, at the very least, a capable replacement for conventional catheter-based pH monitoring.[36]

Finally, wireless pH testing provides the opportunity for prolonged monitoring. Conventional catheter-based pH monitoring has traditionally evaluated 24 hours of esophageal acid exposure; however, the wireless pH system routinely records up to 48 hours of data. Substantial day-to-day variability in esophageal acid exposure is not uncommon, and the addition of a second 24-hour recording period has been shown to increase the overall sensitivity of the study.[33] In addition, prolonged recording periods may be of particular benefit in the analysis of symptom correlation, especially when symptoms are atypical or infrequent.[37-39] Several studies have also looked at prolonged wireless pH testing using a 96-hour protocol, whereby 2 device receivers are calibrated for the same probe and employed in consecutive 48-hour studies.[23-27] Using this technique allowed for increased detection of acid exposure, enhanced symptom association measurements and assessment of acid exposure, and symptom response both on and off PPI therapy. However, 15% of patients had early capsule detachment and 2 separate receivers were required for each study. Reportedly, future iterations of the wireless pH capsule may allow for prolonged 96-hour monitoring using a single receiver.[40]

There are also disadvantages with the wireless pH system that are important to note. Perhaps the biggest limitation is that the system only records pH. There are increasing data to suggest that nonacid reflux is of clinical importance and a wireless pH system has no means to detect any reflux with a pH greater than 4. In addition, as there is only one recording point, there are no means to assess directionality of bolus flow, making it impossible to distinguish a reflux event from a swallow unless the patient has meticulously entered his or her symptom diary.

A second limitation is cost. The capsule itself is more expensive than a conventional pH catheter; moreover, placement of the probe is usually done under the guise of endoscopy, and this significantly increases the total cost yet further. To avoid this issue, it is possible to place the wireless pH probe transorally using manometric landmarks and a conversion factor of 4 cm. In a study by Lacy and colleagues, 308 patients underwent unsedated transoral placement of a wireless pH probe based on manometric landmarks. No complications were reported, and only 3 patients (< 1%) were unable to tolerate transoral unsedated placement.[41] However, this method of placement is not the standard at most institutions at present.

Possible patient discomfort is another potential drawback with the wireless pH system. In the initial publication regarding wireless pH testing, 10 of 29 patients recorded esophageal discomfort (35%) with 2 patients requiring endoscopic probe removal due to these symptoms.[33] Similar rates of chest discomfort and foreign body sensation have been described by other investigators.[31,32] However, in other studies, the rates of chest pain and foreign body sensation are significantly higher, though the symptoms were largely viewed as mild and the patients were able to complete the study.[30,42] Endoscopic removal of the probe has been reported to be necessary in approximately 2% of patients due to severe symptoms.[43]

Finally, another potential drawback of the wireless pH system is inadequate data collection. The recording efficacy of wireless pH monitoring appears to be greater than 95%; however, if early capsule detachment does occur, it may not be noted until after the data are downloaded, and the study may need to be repeated, which increases cost and patient inconvenience. In addition, if the capsule does dislodge and leave the esophagus but recording continues, the interpreter may derive an erroneous conclusion regarding esophageal acid exposure. While most cases of early detachment can be detected by the characteristic presence of prolonged gastric acid exposure, in the context of achlorhydria (either physiological or medication induced) this interpretation may be challenging. Finally, if the patient is too far away from the recorder, prolonged lapses in data can occur. As stated above, recording is adequate in over 95% of patients; however, this may be a concern in a subset of patients.

Impedance Testing

The main limitation with pH testing is that it only identifies the presence of acid in the esophagus and does not explain why a patient may have symptoms despite appropriate acid-suppressive therapy. There are considerable data to show that weakly acidic or nonacidic reflux can induce symptoms. It is impossible to adequately evaluate that question with a modality that only measures pH. By assessing intraluminal bolus movement (liquid and gas) independent of pH properties, intraluminal impedance monitoring has the ability to assess both acidic and nonacidic reflux and is the most sensitive means available for ambulatory reflux monitoring at present (Figure 2-1).[44]

Intraluminal impedance monitoring was first described in 1991[45] but has gained increasing attention over the past decade. The basic concept is that different substances in the esophageal lumen (ie, air or liquid) will have different conductive properties. By applying an alternating current through a catheter containing multiple ring electrodes, one can define both intraluminal contents and bolus movement, both in antegrade and

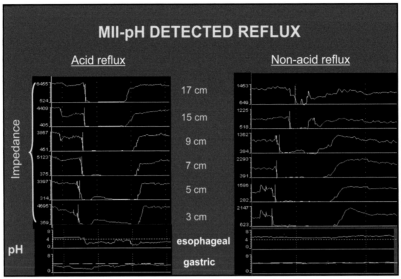

Figure 2-1. Multichannel impedance and pH tracings of 2 reflux episodes recording pH in the stomach (bottom tracing) and distal esophagus (second from bottom) and impedance at 3, 5, 7, 9, 15, and 17 cm above the lower esophageal sphincter. Reflux is identified when the impedance, in ohms, falls to baseline until a swallow restores it back to baseline.

retrograde fashion. If this is then combined with a pH electrode, it is possible to separate acid and nonacid reflux events based on pH information. In addition, reflux events can be separated from swallows based on bolus movement. This may also increase the sensitivity of the study and prevent false-positive interpretations based on food or liquid intake not recorded in the patient diary.

Like other modalities, intraluminal impedance monitoring has clear advantages and disadvantages that are worth discussion. The key advantage is that it allows assessment of weakly acidic or nonacidic reflux, which is not possible with a system limited to pH alone. In the initial report of postprandial impedance monitoring in patients with typical symptoms who had failed PPI therapy, the number of reflux events before and after PPI therapy were similar; however, the pH of the refluxate shifted upward significantly with PPI therapy, and residual symptoms were predominantly linked with nonacid reflux.[46] This finding was supported by Hemmink and colleagues, who evaluated 30 patients with intraluminal impedance monitoring both before and after PPI therapy. They found that the total number and proximal extent of reflux events were unaffected by PPI therapy; however, the bulk of reflux events shifted from acidic to weakly acidic. Similar to the prior report, they also noted symptom correlation with weakly acidic and nonacidic reflux events that would have been missed with pH testing alone.[47]

In patients with continued symptoms despite PPI therapy, there appears to be significant diagnostic gain from the inclusion of intraluminal impedance monitoring. In a study evaluating 168 patients with continued symptoms on twice-daily PPI therapy, 37% had symptomatic nonacid reflux that would not have been recognized by the evaluation of pH alone; whereas, only 11% had failed acid suppression with symptom correlation.[48] Similar results have been reported by other investigators, with the bulk of data suggesting that weakly acidic or nonacidic reflux episodes elicit symptoms in 30% to 40% of patients on PPI therapy.[49-51] This population would be missed entirely if one evaluated reflux via pH alone.

A second advantage of intraluminal impedance monitoring is the ability to separate a swallow from a reflux event. Because impedance allows visualization of bolus flow throughout the esophagus, it has the potential to separate movement based on antegrade and retrograde motion. Agrawal and colleagues demonstrated that commonly ingested substances (eg, coffee, tea, wine, soda, or fruit juice) can transiently decrease the esophageal pH and mimic a reflux event via pH monitoring. While patients are instructed to record all intake on their diary log, it is unclear how often this occurs, and commonly ingested substances that may be sipped throughout the day could easily be forgotten by patients.[52] Further investigation reported that, via this mechanism, the use of pH-only testing would overdiagnose abnormal acid reflux in up to 22% of tested patients.[53] One could then argue that even in the detection of acid reflux, the addition of intraluminal impedance monitoring has added value and improves the specificity of the study.

A third advantage is the ability to detect the proximal extent of reflux. Because most pH studies record at 5 cm proximal to the lower esophageal sphincter, it is impossible to assess proximal reflux extent with standard pH-monitoring equipment. Even with pH-monitoring systems that provide multiple pH sensors, the yield of impedance is still significantly greater as a percentage of reflux events will change from acidic to weakly acidic as the refluxate extends proximally along the esophageal body. In a recent study comparing pH/impedance to multichannel pH testing (3 recording sites), impedance was reported to show a higher sensitivity for the detection of proximal reflux as 30% of acid reflux events became weakly acidic in the proximal recording sites.[54] In addition to increasing diagnostic yield in patients with atypical symptoms (eg, hoarseness and cough), this feature may also be an advantage in assessment of typical symptom correlation given that there is a direct relationship between the proximal extent of reflux and reflux perception.[51]

However, while there are multiple advantages to intraluminal impedance monitoring, there are also some drawbacks that have limited widespread applicability and acceptance of this technology. To begin with, the interpretation of impedance tracings can be time consuming and require training and expertise.[55-57] The automated interpretation software may overestimate the number of reflux events, and manual interpretation of the tracings is still required.[58] Interpretation may be especially difficult or even impossible in patients with low impedance baselines, which is often seen in Barrett's esophagus. These factors may pose a challenge for busy clinicians, who may not have the time for training and interpretation. This is in contrast to pH monitoring, which is relatively straightforward and easily performed in a community practice setting.

A second limitation is the need for an indwelling 24-hour nasogastric catheter. With the advent of wireless pH monitoring, many patients are aware of the wireless options and prefer to avoid a catheter-based study. There are also data to suggest that patients may limit reflux-provoking activities during a catheter-based study, raising concerns that recorded findings may not reflect baseline activity.[28,29] Finally, with current technology, recording is limited to 24 hours, which may be an issue if symptoms are not occurring on a daily basis.

A final limitation of impedance testing is the limited amount of normal data for studies performed on PPI therapy. Three independent multicenter studies have provided normative data for controls undergoing intraluminal impedance monitoring without acid suppression.[59-61] However, intraluminal impedance studies are commonly performed on PPI therapy and normative data regarding those studies are not well established. As there have been multiple studies suggesting that PPI use does not change the number of reflux events (rather, only the pH of the refluxate),[46,47] one could argue that the same normative data described for normal subjects off of PPI therapy holds for patients on medications. Data from our laboratory suggest that normative values for patients on PPI therapy should not exceed 48 reflux episodes per 24 hours.[62]

THE ROLE OF NONACID REFLUX

While there is agreement that impedance is the most sensitive method available to detect reflux and that a significant percentage of PPI nonresponders will have symptomatic nonacid reflux on intraluminal impedance monitoring (30% to 40%), there is controversy as to whether the detection of nonacidic reflux is of clinical significance.[57,63,64] However, there are several small studies that suggest that the detection of symptomatic nonacid reflux may significantly impact clinical outcomes.

Mainie and colleagues evaluated 19 patients referred to laparoscopic Nissen fundoplication after undergoing intraluminal impedance monitoring. With impedance, 18 of 19 patients on PPI therapy demonstrated a positive symptom index. After surgery, 16 of the 17 patients with a positive preoperative symptom index and follow-up data were asymptomatic or markedly improved. In this study, 11 of the 19 patients did have prior documentation of reflux by either pH monitoring or endoscopy; however, 8 patients did not have prior documentation of abnormal pH exposure and would fall under the label of symptomatic nonacid reflux.[65]

A second small study from Switzerland evaluated the role of intraluminal impedance monitoring in patients undergoing fundoplication and reported that, in the 12 patients studied, intraluminal impedance monitoring improved the pre- and postoperative assessment of reflux patients and resulted in a higher symptom-reflux association. In this study, only 3 of 12 patients had a positive symptom index prior to surgery using pH data alone; however, when intraluminal impedance monitoring was added to the equation, the symptom index was positive in 11 of the 12 patients. Antireflux surgery was reported to be successful in 11 of the 12 patients, and without the additional information that impedance provided, the majority of the patients in this study would not have qualified for surgery.[66]

In a third study, Tutuian and colleagues evaluated the role of intraluminal impedance monitoring in chronic cough despite acid-suppressive therapy. In the evaluation of 50 patients, 13 (26%) were found with a positive symptom index on intraluminal impedance monitoring. Six of these patients underwent fundoplication with cessation of cough recorded in all.[67]

In a fourth study, an Italian group prospectively followed 314 consecutive patients who underwent pH/impedance monitoring for refractory reflux. Of this group, 62 patients underwent laparoscopic fundoplication. Seventeen patients (27.4%) had normal pH values with abnormal reflux numbers on impedance, and 12 patients (19.3%) had normal pH with an abnormal symptom index on pH/impedance. The investigators reported 98% patient satisfaction following the procedure and also reported that the data from intraluminal impedance monitoring allowed them to extend the option of surgery to an additional 40% of patients who underwent investigation but had negative pH data.[68]

While these data are limited and the numbers of patients reported are relatively small, the conclusion of each study is identical: symptomatic nonacid reflux is clinically significant and modification of that reflux (in these reports via surgery) leads to improved quality of life. More outcome studies are needed, especially with regard to medical therapy of nonacid reflux; however, given the limited data above, it does seem that symptomatic nonacid reflux is an important clinical category to distinguish and any investigation regarding refractory reflux symptoms needs to account for this entity.

Considering all of the above, we prefer monitoring reflux using catheter-based impedance pH while continuing with acid-suppressive therapy. This approach will provide the most information to resolve why the patient is having symptoms despite such therapy.

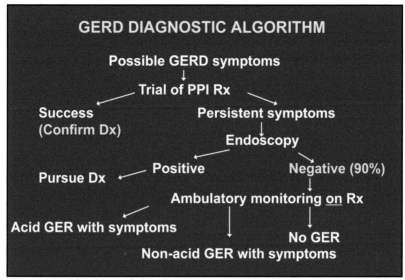

Figure 2-2. Algorithm of the diagnostic approach to patients with suspected GERD symptoms, indicating the preference for testing with ambulatory impedance-pH monitoring while continuing the PPI therapy.

CONCLUSION

GERD is an important clinical entity. Given the significant number of patients affected and the availability of over-the-counter PPI use, refractory GERD is now the most common presentation of reflux to gastroenterologists. In the context of incomplete symptom relief and/or warning signs, endoscopic evaluation is usually the first step, although diagnostic yield of this approach is relatively low, particularly considering the widespread use of empiric PPI therapy. Ambulatory pH testing has traditionally been the next diagnostic test performed and is worth consideration in select patients, especially given the widespread availability and ease of interpretation. Over the past decade, symptomatic nonacid reflux has emerged as a clinically important entity, accounting for 30% to 40% of refractory GERD patients. Intraluminal impedance monitoring is the gold standard to evaluate nonacid reflux and should be considered in all patients with refractory symptoms and an unclear diagnosis despite PPI therapy. Our suggested algorithms for evaluation of typical GERD are detailed in Figures 2-2 and 2-3.

REFERENCES

1. Shaheen NJ, Hansen RA, Morgan DR, et al. The burden of gastrointestinal and liver diseases, 2006. *Am J Gastroenterol.* 2006;101:2128-2138.
2. Locke GR 3rd, Talley NJ, Fett SL, Zinsmeister AR, Melton LJ 3rd. Prevalence and clinical spectrum of gastroesophageal reflux: a population-based study in Olmsted County, Minnesota. *Gastroenterology.* 1997;112:1448-1456.
3. Vakil N, van Zanten SV, Kahrilas P, Dent J, Jones R. The Montreal definition and classification of gastroesophageal reflux disease: a global evidence-based consensus. *Am J Gastroenterol.* 2006;101:1900-1920; quiz 43.
4. Kahrilas PJ, Shaheen NJ, Vaezi MF. American Gastroenterological Association Institute technical review on the management of gastroesophageal reflux disease. *Gastroenterology.* 2008;135:1392-1413, e1-e5.

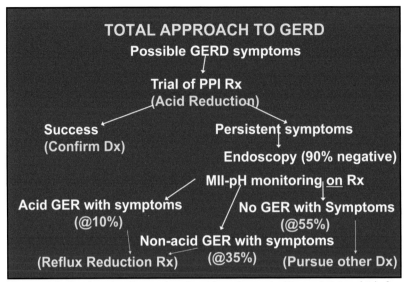

Figure 2-3. Further details on the algorithm shown in Figure 2-2 in which frequency of findings during testing are shown and suggestions for possible therapy are indicated.

5. DeVault KR, Castell DO. Updated guidelines for the diagnosis and treatment of gastroesophageal reflux disease. *Am J Gastroenterol.* 2005;100:190-200.
6. Hirano I, Richter JE. ACG practice guidelines: esophageal reflux testing. *Am J Gastroenterol.* 2007;102:668-685.
7. Kahrilas PJ, Shaheen NJ, Vaezi MF, et al. American Gastroenterological Association medical position statement on the management of gastroesophageal reflux disease. *Gastroenterology.* 2008;135:1383-1391, e1-e5.
8. Pandolfino JE, Vela MF. Esophageal-reflux monitoring. *Gastrointest Endosc.* 2009;69:917-930, e1.
9. Gonsalves N, Kahrilas PJ. Eosinophilic oesophagitis in adults. *Neurogastroenterol Motil.* 2009;21:1017-1026.
10. Liacouras CA. Eosinophilic esophagitis. *Gastroenterol Clin North Am.* 2008;37:989-998, xi.
11. Furuta GT, Liacouras CA, Collins MH, et al. Eosinophilic esophagitis in children and adults: a systematic review and consensus recommendations for diagnosis and treatment. *Gastroenterology.* 2007;133:1342-1363.
12. Spechler SJ, Genta RM, Souza RF. Thoughts on the complex relationship between gastroesophageal reflux disease and eosinophilic esophagitis. *Am J Gastroenterol.* 2007;102:1301-1306.
13. Richter JE. The patient with refractory gastroesophageal reflux disease. *Dis Esophagus.* 2006;19:443-447.
14. Lichtenstein DR, Cash BD, Davila R, et al. Role of endoscopy in the management of GERD. *Gastrointest Endosc.* 2007;66:219-224.
15. Richter JE. Diagnostic tests for gastroesophageal reflux disease. *Am J Med Sci.* 2003;326:300-308.
16. Moayyedi P, Talley NJ. Gastro-oesophageal reflux disease. *Lancet.* 2006;367:2086-2100.
17. Ronkainen J, Aro P, Storskrubb T, et al. High prevalence of gastroesophageal reflux symptoms and esophagitis with or without symptoms in the general adult Swedish population: a Kalixanda study report. *Scand J Gastroenterol.* 2005;40:275-285.
18. Poh CH, Gasiorowska A, Navarro-Rodriguez T, et al. Upper GI tract findings in patients with heartburn in whom proton pump inhibitor treatment failed versus those not receiving antireflux treatment. *Gastrointest Endosc.* 2010;71:28-34.
19. Gerson LB. Diagnostic yield of upper endoscopy in treated GERD patients. *Gastroenterology.* 2010;139:1408-1409.
20. Rath HC, Timmer A, Kunkel C, et al. Comparison of interobserver agreement for different scoring systems for reflux esophagitis: impact of level of experience. *Gastrointest Endosc.* 2004;60:44-49.
21. Gonsalves N, Policarpio-Nicolas M, Zhang Q, Rao MS, Hirano I. Histopathologic variability and endoscopic correlates in adults with eosinophilic esophagitis. *Gastrointest Endosc.* 2006;64:313-319.

22. Dellon ES, Gibbs WB, Fritchie KJ, et al. Clinical, endoscopic, and histologic findings distinguish eosin-ophilic esophagitis from gastroesophageal reflux disease. *Clin Gastroenterol Hepatol.* 2009;7:1305-1313; quiz 261.

23. Calabrese C, Liguori G, Gabusi V, et al. Ninety-six-hour wireless oesophageal pH monitoring following proton pump inhibitor administration in NERD patients. *Aliment Pharmacol Ther.* 2008;28:250-255.

24. Scarpulla G, Camilleri S, Galante P, Manganaro M, Fox M. The impact of prolonged pH measurements on the diagnosis of gastroesophageal reflux disease: 4-day wireless pH studies. *Am J Gastroenterol.* 2007;102:2642-2647.

25. Hirano I, Zhang Q, Pandolfino JE, Kahrilas PJ. Four-day Bravo pH capsule monitoring with and with-out proton pump inhibitor therapy. *Clin Gastroenterol Hepatol.* 2005;3:1083-1088.

26. Garrean CP, Zhang Q, Gonsalves N, Hirano I. Acid reflux detection and symptom-reflux asso-ciation using 4-day wireless pH recording combining 48-hour periods off and on PPI therapy. *Am J Gastroenterol.* 2008;103:1631-1637.

27. Sweis R, Fox M, Anggiansah A, Wong T. Prolonged, wireless pH-studies have a high diagnostic yield in patients with reflux symptoms and negative 24-h catheter-based pH-studies. *Neurogastroenterol Motil.* 2011;23(5):419-426.

28. Mearin F, Balboa A, Dot J, Maldonado O, Malagelada JR. How standard is a standard day during a standard ambulatory 24-hour esophageal pH monitoring? *Scand J Gastroenterol.* 1998;33:583-585.

29. Fass R, Hell R, Sampliner RE, et al. Effect of ambulatory 24-hour esophageal pH monitoring on reflux-provoking activities. *Dig Dis Sci.* 1999;44:2263-2269.

30. Bradley AG, Crowell MD, DiBaise JK, et al. Comparison of the impact of wireless versus catheter-based pH-metry on daily activities and study-related symptoms. *J Clin Gastroenterol.* 2011;45:100-106.

31. Wong WM, Bautista J, Dekel R, et al. Feasibility and tolerability of transnasal/per-oral placement of the wireless pH capsule vs. traditional 24-h oesophageal pH monitoring—a randomized trial. *Aliment Pharmacol Ther.* 2005;21:155-163.

32. Grigolon A, Bravi I, Cantu P, Conte D, Penagini R. Wireless pH monitoring: better tolerability and lower impact on daily habits. *Dig Liver Dis.* 2007;39:720-724.

33. Pandolfino JE, Richter JE, Ours T, Guardino JM, Chapman J, Kahrilas PJ. Ambulatory esophageal pH monitoring using a wireless system. *Am J Gastroenterol.* 2003;98:740-749.

34. Sweis R, Fox M, Anggiansah R, et al. Patient acceptance and clinical impact of Bravo monitoring in patients with previous failed catheter-based studies. *Aliment Pharmacol Ther.* 2009;29:669-676.

35. Pandolfino JE, Schreiner MA, Lee TJ, Zhang Q, Boniquit C, Kahrilas PJ. Comparison of the Bravo wire-less and Digitrapper catheter-based pH monitoring systems for measuring esophageal acid exposure. *Am J Gastroenterol.* 2005;100:1466-1476.

36. Pandolfino JE, Kwiatek MA. Use and utility of the Bravo pH capsule. *J Clin Gastroenterol.* 2008;42:571-578.

37. Clouse RE, Prakash C, Haroian L. Symptom association tests are improved by the extended ambulatory pH recording time with the Bravo capsule. *Gastroenterology.* 2003;124:A537.

38. Pandolfino JE, Kahrilas PJ. Prolonged pH monitoring: Bravo capsule. *Gastrointest Endosc Clin N Am.* 2005;15:307-318.

39. Prakash C, Clouse RE. Value of extended recording time with wireless pH monitoring in evaluating gastroesophageal reflux disease. *Clin Gastroenterol Hepatol.* 2005;3:329-334.

40. Gawron AJ, Hirano I. Advances in diagnostic testing for gastroesophageal reflux disease. *World J Gastroenterol.* 2010;16:3750-3756.

41. Lacy BE, O'Shana T, Hynes M, et al. Safety and tolerability of transoral Bravo capsule placement after transnasal manometry using a validated conversion factor. *Am J Gastroenterol.* 2007;102:24-32.

42. Ahlawat SK, Novak DJ, Williams DC, Maher KA, Barton F, Benjamin SB. Day-to-day variability in acid reflux patterns using the Bravo pH monitoring system. *J Clin Gastroenterol.* 2006;40:20-24.

43. Prakash C, Jonnalagadda S, Azar R, Clouse RE. Endoscopic removal of the wireless pH monitoring capsule in patients with severe discomfort. *Gastrointest Endosc.* 2006;64:828-832.

44. Sifrim D, Castell D, Dent J, Kahrilas PJ. Gastro-oesophageal reflux monitoring: review and consensus report on detection and definitions of acid, non-acid, and gas reflux. *Gut.* 2004;53:1024-1031.

45. Silny J. Intraluminal multiple electric impedance procedure for measurement of gastrointestinal motil-ity. *J Gastrointest Mot.* 1991;3:151-162.

46. Vela MF, Camacho-Lobato L, Srinivasan R, Tutuian R, Katz PO, Castell DO. Simultaneous intraesophageal impedance and pH measurement of acid and nonacid gastroesophageal reflux: effect of omeprazole. *Gastroenterology.* 2001;120:1599-1606.

47. Hemmink GJ, Bredenoord AJ, Weusten BL, Monkelbaan JF, Timmer R, Smout AJ. Esophageal pH-impedance monitoring in patients with therapy-resistant reflux symptoms: 'on' or 'off' proton pump inhibitor? *Am J Gastroenterol.* 2008;103:2446-2453.

48. Mainie I, Tutuian R, Shay S, et al. Acid and non-acid reflux in patients with persistent symptoms despite acid suppressive therapy: a multicentre study using combined ambulatory impedance-pH monitoring. *Gut.* 2006;55:1398-1402.

49. Kline MM, Ewing M, Simpson N, Lainc L. The utility of intraluminal impedance in patients with gastroesophageal reflux disease-like symptoms but normal endoscopy and 24-hour pH testing. *Clin Gastroenterol Hepatol.* 2008;6:880-885; quiz 36.

50. Zerbib F, Roman S, Ropert A, et al. Esophageal pH-impedance monitoring and symptom analysis in GERD: a study in patients off and on therapy. *Am J Gastroenterol.* 2006;101:1956-1963.

51. Zerbib F, Duriez A, Roman S, Capdepont M, Mion F. Determinants of gastro-oesophageal reflux perception in patients with persistent symptoms despite proton pump inhibitors. *Gut.* 2008;57:156-160.

52. Agrawal A, Tutuian R, Hila A, Freeman J, Castell DO. Ingestion of acidic foods mimics gastroesophageal reflux during pH monitoring. *Dig Dis Sci.* 2005;50:1916-1920.

53. Hila A, Agrawal A, Castell DO. Combined multichannel intraluminal impedance and pH esophageal testing compared to pH alone for diagnosing both acid and weakly acidic gastroesophageal reflux. *Clin Gastroenterol Hepatol.* 2007;5:172-177.

54. Emerenziani S, Ribolsi M, Sifrim D, Blondeau K, Cicala M. Regional oesophageal sensitivity to acid and weakly acidic reflux in patients with non-erosive reflux disease. *Neurogastroenterol Motil.* 2009;21:253-258.

55. Shay S. Esophageal impedance monitoring: the ups and downs of a new test. *Am J Gastroenterol.* 2004;99:1020-1022.

56. Park W, Vaezi MF. Esophageal impedance recording: clinical utility and limitations. *Curr Gastroenterol Rep.* 2005;7:182-189.

57. Richter JE. Con: impedance-pH testing does not commonly alter management of GERD. *Am J Gastroenterol.* 2009;104:2667-2669.

58. Roman S, Bruley des Varannes S, Pouderoux P, et al. Ambulatory 24-h oesophageal impedance-pH recordings: reliability of automatic analysis for gastro-oesophageal reflux assessment. *Neurogastroenterol Motil.* 2006;18:978-986.

59. Shay S, Tutuian R, Sifrim D, et al. Twenty-four hour ambulatory simultaneous impedance and pH monitoring: a multicenter report of normal values from 60 healthy volunteers. *Am J Gastroenterol.* 2004;99:1037-1043.

60. Zerbib F, des Varannes SB, Roman S, et al. Normal values and day-to-day variability of 24-h ambulatory oesophageal impedance-pH monitoring in a Belgian-French cohort of healthy subjects. *Aliment Pharmacol Ther.* 2005;22:1011-1021.

61. Zentilin P, Iiritano E, Dulbecco P, et al. Normal values of 24-h ambulatory intraluminal impedance combined with pH-metry in subjects eating a Mediterranean diet. *Dig Liver Dis.* 2006;38:226-232.

62. Tutuian R, Mainie I, Agrawal A, Freeman J, Castell DO. Normal values for ambulatory 24-hour combined impedance-pH monitoring on acid suppressive therapy. *Gastroenterology.* 2006;130:A171.

63. Blondeau K, Tack J. Pro: impedance testing is useful in the management of GERD. *Am J Gastroenterol.* 2009;104:2664-2666.

64. Shay S. A balancing view: impedance-pH testing in gerd-limited role for now, perhaps more helpful in the future. *Am J Gastroenterol.* 2009;104:2669-2670.

65. Mainie I, Tutuian R, Agrawal A, Adams D, Castell DO. Combined multichannel intraluminal impedance-pH monitoring to select patients with persistent gastro-oesophageal reflux for laparoscopic Nissen fundoplication. *Br J Surg.* 2006;93:1483-1487.

66. Gruebel C, Linke G, Tutuian R, et al. Prospective study examining the impact of multichannel intraluminal impedance on antireflux surgery. *Surg Endosc.* 2008;22:1241-1247.

67. Tutuian R, Mainie I, Agrawal A, Adams D, Castell DO. Nonacid reflux in patients with chronic cough on acid-suppressive therapy. *Chest.* 2006;130:386-391.

68. del Genio G, Tolone S, del Genio F, et al. Prospective assessment of patient selection for antireflux surgery by combined multichannel intraluminal impedance pH monitoring. *J Gastrointest Surg.* 2008;12:1491-1496.

chapter 3

Pulmonary Manifestations of GERD

Controversies and Consensus

Lindsey B. Roenigk, MD and Susan M. Harding, MD

Since the 12th century, physicians have noted that gastroesophageal reflux (GER) symptoms are temporally associated with respiratory symptoms.[1] GER causes cough, triggers asthma, and can impact other pulmonary diseases.[2] Recent data provide further insight into the association of GER and pulmonary disease.

PATHOPHYSIOLOGICAL MECHANISMS OF GASTROESOPHAGEAL REFLUX-INDUCED PULMONARY DISEASE

The lung and the esophagus share common embryonic foregut origins and vagal innervation.[2] Esophageal acid initiates vagally mediated reflexes, resulting in bronchoconstriction.[3,4] Local axonal reflexes also provide a direct connection between the esophagus and the lung and are activated in the esophagus.[5] Esophageal acid can also serve as a primer for heightened bronchial reactivity to bronchoconstrictive triggers.[6] Microaspiration of acid into the upper airway stimulates a much greater bronchoconstrictive response than acid in the esophagus.[7,8] Esophageal acid and gastric contents also initiate the release of neuroinflammatory mediators in the airway.[9] Lastly, bronchoconstriction increases the frequency of transient lower esophageal sphincter relaxations (TLESR), predisposing it to more GER events.[10] Table 3-1 reviews these and other potential mechanisms.

DiMarino AJ Jr, Cohen S, eds.
Extraesophageal Manifestations of GERD (pp 35-48).
© 2013 Taylor & Francis Group.

Table 3-1	Mechanisms of Interaction Between the Esophagus and the Lung	
	POINT	**COUNTERPOINT**
Vagal reflex	In a dog model, esophageal acid-induced bronchoconstriction; these findings have been reproduced in humans.[3]	Bronchoconstriction resulted in a modest reduction in peak expiratory flow rates without reduction in forced expiratory volume over 1 second.[4]
Local axonal reflexes	Evidence suggests a direct connection between the esophagus and trachea without input from higher cortical structures.[5]	This evidence is in animal models, not humans.
Heightened bronchial reactivity	Data suggest esophageal acid primes the lungs for an exaggerated response to triggers.[6]	Eradicating GER does not cure the underlying pulmonary disease.
Microaspiration	Compared to acid in the esophagus, acid in the upper airway elicits changes in pulmonary function that are orders of magnitude higher in humans.[7]	The vagus nerve also plays a role in microaspiration in a cat model.[8]
GER-initiated inflammation	Neuroinflammatory and oxidative stress biomarkers are triggered by GER in the lung.[9]	Data suggest that these mechanisms can alter the pathophysiology of the lung disease.
Bronchoconstriction-induced GER events	Methacholine-induced bronchoconstriction lowers lower esophageal sphincter pressure and induces GER events.[10]	A mechanism may exist allowing methacholine to directly affect lower esophageal sphincter pressure.

Bottom Line

Multiple avenues for physiological interaction exist between the lungs and the esophagus that allow GER to alter lung physiology, thus leading to disease states.

GASTROESOPHAGEAL REFLUX AND ASTHMA

Asthma is an airway disease resulting in bronchoconstriction and inflammation that is initiated by multiple triggers. Triggers can vary from patient to patient, and a single patient is often susceptible to multiple triggers. GER is a potential asthma trigger and coexists in up to 80% of asthma patients.[11] Potentially, GER therapy may improve asthma outcomes in selected patients. There are data to both support and disprove this assertion.

Gastroesophageal Reflux Epidemiology in Asthma Patients

Asthma patients have an increased risk of developing GER compared to nonasthmatics, even when controlling for confounders.[12] A study of 101,366 veterans with esophagitis showed that these veterans had an increased likelihood of developing asthma with an odds ratio of 1.51 (95% confidence interval [CI] 1.43 to 1.59) compared to controls.[13] GER prevalence in asthma patients ranges between 34% and 89%.[2] Sontag et al found that 82% of asthma patients had abnormal esophageal acid contact times on esophageal pH monitoring.[11] In 186 consecutive asthma patients, they found that 43% had esophagitis or Barrett's esophagus.[14] Field et al found heartburn to be present in 77% of asthma patients, compared to 50% of controls. Also, 41% of asthma patients had GER-associated pulmonary symptoms, and 28% had used their rescue inhalers during a GER episode.[15] We showed that 79% of respiratory symptoms were temporally related to esophageal acid events in asthma patients with GER.[16] Furthermore, in consecutive asthma patients without GER symptoms, 65% had abnormal esophageal acid contact times.[17] Thus, GER may be clinically silent in many asthma patients.

Asthma patients have risk factors that predispose them to GER development. Bronchoconstriction and airflow obstruction increase the thoraco-abdominal pressure gradient and increase the frequency of TLESR, both of which promote GER. Asthma medications (eg, albuterol, steroids, and theophylline) also predispose to GER development.[18]

Testing and Diagnosis

Currently, no diagnostic test is available to identify asthma patients with GER therapy-responsive asthma. Barium esophagram, esophageal manometry and pH monitoring, endoscopy, exhaled breath condensate (EBC) pH analysis, and sputum for lipid-laden macrophages and other biomarkers do not correctly identify these patients.

Esophageal pH monitoring offers the ability to correlate asthma symptoms with GER events, to diagnose silent GER, and to assess for adequacy of acid suppression in patients on GER medications.[2] Abnormal amounts of proximal esophageal acid exposure potentially predict asthma improvement.[19] Proximal esophageal acid exposure in asthma patients with asymptomatic GER is associated with lower asthma quality of life; however, its presence did not impact lower airway function.[20] Combining esophageal pH with impedance monitoring can identify nonacid reflux, but the role of nonacid reflux in asthma is largely unknown.

Since GER is highly prevalent in asthma patients and there is no diagnostic test that identifies GER-therapy responsive asthma, widespread testing for GER does not have clinical utility. It is our opinion that the best current diagnostic test for identifying GER therapy-responsive asthma is a 3-month empiric trial of pharmacologic acid suppression with twice-daily proton pump inhibitors (PPIs) in asthma patients with GER symptoms.[2] Prospective studies are needed to evaluate this method's diagnostic accuracy.

Treatment

Asthma therapy should be guided by the clinical practice guidelines outlined by the National Asthma Education and Prevention Program published in 2007.[21] Although not examined in placebo-controlled trials, behavioral and GER lifestyle changes should be implemented in asthma patients with GER symptoms. Medical GER therapy improves asthma outcomes in selected asthma patients with GER symptoms. Fundoplication for an asthma indication should be reserved for patients who have asthma improvement on medical GER therapy.

Asthma Outcomes With Gastroesophageal Reflux Therapy

In 2003, a Cochrane Database review of 12 randomized, controlled trials of medical GER therapy and asthma was published.[22] Half of these trials used PPIs. Nine of the 12 trials reported a significant improved asthma outcome, but there was no interstudy consistency in which outcome was affected. However, subgroups of asthma patients might benefit from GER therapy.[22]

Since 2004, 5 double-blind, placebo-controlled trials utilizing PPI therapy for an adequate duration were reported. The American Lung Association Asthma Clinical Research Centers (ALA-ACRC) reported the results of its randomized trial of twice-daily esomeprazole for 24 weeks in 412 inadequately controlled asthma patients without GER symptoms.[23] The primary outcome was a reduction of Type I episodes of poor asthma control (definition: reduction of morning peak expiratory flow [PEF] by > 30%, urgent office visits associated with asthma symptoms, or need for oral corticosteroids). Secondary outcomes included pulmonary function, asthma symptoms, nocturnal asthma symptoms, and quality of life; no difference was noted in any of these outcomes. Thus, asthma patients without GER symptoms are unlikely to benefit from medical GER therapy.[23]

Littner et al examined outcomes in 207 moderate to severe asthma patients with GER symptoms using lansoprazole 30 mg twice daily or placebo twice daily for 24 weeks.[24] Significant improvement occurred in the treated group in the emotional function domain of the Asthma Quality of Life Questionnaire Score. A post-hoc analysis noted that the PPI group had a significant reduction in acute asthma exacerbations and a prolonged time to first asthma exacerbation. There was no significant change in asthma medication use, pulmonary function, or asthma symptoms.[24]

Kiljander et al examined 770 moderate to severe asthma patients with placebo or esomeprazole 40 mg twice daily for 16 weeks.[25] Patients with GER and nocturnal asthma symptoms had statistically significant improvement in PEF rate (8.7 L/min, p = 0.03) and in evening PEF (10.2 L/min, p = 0.012). While these findings reach statistical significance, the clinical significance of a PEF increase of 8.7 L/min and 10.2 L/min is questionable.[25] Asthma patients without GER symptoms did not have improvement in PEF, confirming the findings of the ALA-ACRC study.

Kiljander et al also reported a separate group of 828 patients with moderate to severe asthma and GER symptoms, randomized to receive either 26 weeks of placebo or esomeprazole 40 mg once or twice daily, with morning PEF as the primary outcome. Both active treatment groups had improvement in morning PEF, forced expiratory volume (FEV_1), and asthma quality of life measures, although these improvements were modest.[26]

Thus, not all asthma patients warrant an empiric medical GER treatment trial, but it suggests that some subgroups (eg, asthma patients with GER symptoms) could benefit from therapy. A key unanswered question is: What are the predictors for asthma improvement? Potential predictors noted in previous studies include difficult to control asthma, nonallergic asthma, nocturnal asthma, obesity, proximal acid GER, weekly regurgitation, and reflux-associated asthma symptoms (Table 3-2).[2,19]

Surgical trials examining asthma outcomes have study design flaws. A 1999 review identified 417 asthma patients undergoing fundoplication, with 90% reporting improvement in GER symptoms. Asthma symptoms and medication use decreased by 79% and 88%, respectively, but only 27% of subjects had improved pulmonary function.[27]

Two studies compared medical therapy, surgical therapy, or placebo in asthmatics with GER. Larrain et al followed 81 intrinsic asthmatics who were randomized to either placebo, cimetidine (4 times a day), or surgical therapy.[28] The cimetidine and surgical groups had similar rates of improvement in pulmonary function and asthma medication use.[28] Sontag et al randomized 62 patients to receive ranitidine 3 times a day, fundoplication, or antacids

Table 3-2	**Potential Predictors of Asthma Response**
ASTHMA CHARACTERISTICS	**GASTROESOPHAGEAL REFLUX CHARACTERISTICS**
1. Difficult to control asthma	1. Reflux-associated respiratory symptoms
2. Nonallergic, intrinsic asthma	2. Regurgitation more than once weekly
3. Nocturnal asthma	3. Proximal acid on pH testing
4. Obesity (body mass index > 29.7)	4. Distal acid on pH testing

Reprinted with permission from Harding SM. Gastroesophageal reflux: a potential asthma trigger. *Immunol Allergy Clin N Am.* 2005;25:131-148. Published by Elsevier.

Table 3-3	**Gastroesophageal Reflux and Asthma**	
	POINT	**COUNTERPOINT**
Prevalence and pathophysiology	GER is common in asthmatics.[2]	Asthma and asthma medications may predispose to GER.[2,17]
Diagnosis	No diagnostic test identifies asthmatics who will respond to GER therapy.	Empiric medical GER therapy for 3 months while accessing asthma outcomes is the best way to identify potential responders.[2]
Treatment	Selected asthmatics with GER symptoms will improve with GER therapy.[21-23]	Placebo-controlled trials show that asthmatics without GER symptoms do not have asthma improvement with PPI.[21]
Surgery	Fundoplication for asthma should be considered only in asthma patients who improve with medical GER therapy.[2]	If fundoplication is being considered, careful evaluation of GER should include esophageal manometry and pH and impedance monitoring.[2]

(control). After 2 years, overall asthma status was improved in 75% of the individuals in the surgical group, 9% in the ranitidine group, and 4% in the antacid group.[29]

Controversies

Despite our understanding of pathophysiological mechanisms, many clinical issues remain unresolved. No test accurately predicts which asthma patients respond to PPI therapy. The patient characteristics that respond to GER therapy are unclear. A consensus on how to define a positive response to therapy is also not clearly defined. Some experts say a positive response should be defined as improved asthma symptoms; some argue for more concrete evidence such as improved pulmonary function, PEF, or a reduction in required asthma maintenance medications. We also lack experimental data to support our above position on how to chronically treat GER in asthma patients. Which patients should be referred to surgery and when to refer to surgery are areas needing further investigation. Cost-effectiveness data to compare long-term PPI use to surgery may also contribute to determining the future role of surgery in these patients. All of these issues highlight the need for more large-scale, placebo-controlled trials in the area of GER and asthma (Table 3-3).

Bottom Line

Asthma patients with GER symptoms should empirically receive a 3-month trial of twice-daily PPI therapy. A lack of asthma response at 3 months, defined by any of the mentioned criteria, suggests the patient's asthma is not triggered by GER. In nonresponders, consider 24-hour pH monitoring and/or impedance monitoring to confirm adequate GER control. In patients who do improve, we would suggest tapering the PPIs to daily dosing once asthma improvement plateaus. We would also consider empiric PPI therapy in difficult to control asthma patients, particularly those requiring chronic oral corticosteroids, even in the absence of GER symptoms, although this is more controversial.

GASTROESOPHAGEAL REFLUX AND CHRONIC COUGH

Chronic cough, defined as a cough lasting more than 8 weeks, is one of the most common complaints for which patients seek medical attention, and GER is a common cause of chronic cough.[30] Approximately 10% of chronic cough patients have GER symptoms. *GER-related cough* is defined as cough that responds to GER therapy. GER may be silent in up to 75% of patients with GER-related cough, making its diagnosis much more difficult![31]

Causes of Chronic Cough

Determining the etiology of chronic cough is a diagnostic challenge, as more than 30 causes have been identified. In addition, patients frequently have more than one cause of cough.[31] Cough has been attributable to 2 causes in 18% to 62% of patients and 3 or more causes in up to 42% of patients.[31] So, for cough resolution, all potential causes need to be treated. In an immunocompetent nonsmoker with a normal chest radiograph who does not take an angiotensin converting enzyme (ACE) inhibitor, the 5 most common causes of chronic cough are upper airway cough syndrome (previously noted as postnasal drip syndrome), GER, asthma, eosinophilic bronchitis, and postinfectious cough.[32,33] GER has been estimated to be the cause of cough in 21% to 41% of cases.[31] There are data showing that nonacid reflux also causes cough.[34] So, medications that inhibit gastric acid secretion may not be adequate to treat some patients. The multifactorial etiology of chronic cough is just one of the potential diagnostic pitfalls associated with the management of chronic cough.

Testing and Diagnosis

There is no test or procedure currently able to determine which chronic cough patients will respond to GER medical therapy. The same tests used to evaluate for GER and GER-related asthma are available for GER-related cough, with the addition of tussigenic challenging.[32] Barium esophagrams have a sensitivity of 48% and a specificity of 75% for diagnosing GER-related cough.[35] Twenty-four hour esophageal pH monitoring with cough correlation has become the gold standard for diagnosing GER-related cough; it has a sensitivity of 90% to 100% and specificity of 60% to 100%.[35] The diagnostic test recommended by the American College of Chest Physicians and the British Thoracic Society clinical practice guidelines is an empiric trial of medical GER therapy for 1 to 3 months in chronic cough patients with GER symptoms or in those who are likely to have silent GER.[30,36] Irwin identified a clinical profile of individuals with GER-related cough who did not report esophageal symptoms. This profile includes a chronic cough patient who is a nonsmoker without a history of irritant exposure, who is not on an ACE inhibitor, has a normal or stable chest roentgenograph, and asthma, upper airway cough syndrome, and nonasthmatic eosinophilic bronchitis have been ruled out or has not improved on disease-specific therapy.[30]

Only after the empiric trial fails do they recommend more objective GER testing to evaluate for potential causes of failure.[30] Poe and Kallay examined this approach in a 2003 trial of 214 patients with chronic cough. They were able to diagnose GER-related cough in 79% of patients, and 86% of the patients had cough improvement within 4 weeks of initiating empiric medical GER therapy.[37] If the empiric trial fails, the next test should be 24-hour esophageal pH monitoring with cough correlation combined with impedance monitoring, if feasible. The symptom association probability can be useful using a 2-minute association window.[38] Simultaneous impedance monitoring allows the correlation of weakly acid or nonacid GER events with cough, especially when the patient is on PPI therapy.[32]

Treatment

All patients with GER-related cough should implement GER lifestyle changes. In addition, we recommend twice-daily PPI therapy for at least 2 months. Cough improvement can occur in as little as 2 weeks, but there are also reports of it taking up to 53 days.[39,40] We recommend PPIs over other GER medications because trials using other acid-suppressive drugs note that it takes a longer time for cough improvement to be evident.[41] The delay in the cough response to PPI therapy represents another potential pitfall in chronic cough management. In addition, the esomeprazole package insert notes that 1% of patients report cough as a side effect of this medication.[42]

Surgical fundoplication for GER-related cough can also be successful. Fundoplication has the advantage of controlling nonacid GER. Currently, it is only recommended for those patients who clearly have GER as the cause of their cough, yet have not responded to maximal GER medical therapy and GER lifestyle changes.[32]

Outcomes

In 2006, a Cochrane Database review examined outcomes data for treatment of GER-related cough.[43] This meta-analysis included 6 studies utilizing PPIs. PPIs did not increase the likelihood of cough resolution compared to placebo, but PPIs did improve cough symptom scores. They stated that there was insufficient evidence to conclude that PPIs are universally beneficial for GER-related cough.[43] Most studies had significant limitations in study design. Only 2 studies exclusively enrolled adults. Many of the studies examined patients with other GER-related symptoms. Also, much of the available data were collected prior to the introduction of PPIs. Significant placebo and time period effects may have confounded the results. The final recommendation was that more randomized, controlled trials utilizing PPIs in GER-related cough need to be performed.[40,43]

Data are available for only 2 prospective, placebo-controlled trials utilizing PPIs in adults with GER-related cough. Ours et al examined 23 patients with chronic cough treated with twice-daily PPIs.[40] There was a 35% response rate in patients who had abnormal esophageal acid contact times on esophageal pH monitoring.[40] Kiljander et al examined 48 patients with chronic cough, of which 29 patients had GER.[44] These 29 patients were randomized to receive daily omeprazole or placebo for 8 weeks in a crossover design. There was a 35% to 57% cough improvement rate with PPI therapy. Concerns were raised about the study design because of possible carryover effect.[44]

Cough outcomes after fundoplication for GER-related cough show good results, but studies were performed in highly selected subjects. One advantage to fundoplication is that it treats both acid and nonacid reflux.[45] Allen and Anvari examined long-term outcomes of 905 patients undergoing laparoscopic fundoplication for GER.[46] Two hundred nine patients reported respiratory symptoms (mainly cough) at the time of surgery. At the 6-month, 2-year, and 5-year follow-up, patients complaining of preoperative cough

Table 3-4	Mechanisms of Interaction Between the Esophagus and the Lung	
	POINT	COUNTERPOINT
Causes	GER is a cause of cough in up to 41% of patients with chronic cough.[30]	In chronic cough patients, up to 62% have 2 causes, up to 42% have 3 causes of cough.[31]
Clinical manifestations	GER is clinically silent in up to 75% of patients with GER-related cough.[30]	Identifying clinical features of patients who do not have GER symptoms but have GER-related cough was described by Irwin et al.[30]
Nonacid GER	Nonacid GER is a cause of GER-related cough.[34]	Combined esophageal pH-impedance monitoring is required to identify nonacid GER.
Testing	Carefully correlate esophageal acid and nonacid events with cough using the symptom association probability with a 2-minute association window.[38]	Patients with GER-related cough may have normal esophageal pH values.[32]
Treatment	An empiric GER therapy trial with twice-daily PPI for 3 months can successfully control 80% of GER-related cough patients.[37]	Careful evaluation is recommended in the cough nonresponders to rule out other causes of cough and document inadequate GER control with combined esophageal pH and impedance prior to recommending fundoplication.[32]

reported cough improvement 83%, 74%, and 71% of the time, respectively. Since results diminished over time, patients should be made aware of this possibility. More long-term outcome data are needed to better determine which patients are appropriate candidates for surgical fundoplication.[46]

Controversies

Fewer debates exist around the topic of GER and chronic cough, but there are still some areas that are yet to be clearly defined. Cost analysis of medical versus surgical therapy could show that surgery is less expensive over the patient's lifetime. The role of endoscopic treatment of GER is yet to be defined, but there are data to suggest that it may be an option.[47] As with asthma and GER, we need more prospective, randomized, controlled trials to guide our treatment of GER-related cough (Table 3-4).

Bottom Line

If a patient has suspected GER-related cough, we recommend an empiric trial of twice-daily PPIs for 1 to 3 months. If the patient's cough responds, the dosing can be decreased to once daily. In cough nonresponders, consider 24-hour esophageal pH monitoring with impedance to confirm acid suppression and to correlate cough with acid or nonacid GER events. Lastly, remember that the cause of cough is often multifactorial, and the patient may require multiple therapies for cough resolution.

GASTROESOPHAGEAL REFLUX-RELATED ASPIRATION

Aspiration of gastric contents into the tracheobronchial tree impacts multiple pulmonary diseases, including pulmonary fibrosis, chronic obstructive lung disease (COPD), cystic fibrosis, and the development of bronchiolitis obliterans syndrome (BOS) in lung transplant recipients.

Pathophysiology

Many mechanisms exist to protect the tracheobronchial tree and pulmonary parenchyma from coming in contact with gastric secretions, including the cough reflex, vagally induced bronchoconstriction, glottis function, bronchial cilia, and bronchial secretions. The effect of the aspirate on the lungs, and the lungs' response depends on many factors, especially the nature of what is aspirated. Patients aspirate nasal and oral secretions, food, gastric contents, bile acids, and other toxic fluids. The lungs' response will also be affected by the volume of the aspirate and the frequency of the aspiration.[48]

Different lung diseases have specific risk factors predisposing to aspiration and its effects. For example, in cystic fibrosis, secretions are difficult to expectorate, making it more difficult to clear aspirated gastric contents. Lung transplant recipients are at risk for vagal nerve injury during surgery, impairing their cough reflex.

Diagnosis

In a patient with risk factors for GER-related aspiration or with symptoms suggesting GER-related aspiration, all of the previously mentioned tests to evaluate GER apply. A key additional component is swallowing function assessment. This usually involves a consultation with a speech therapist, which may include a video fluoroscopic swallowing study or fiber optic swallowing assessment with sensory testing.

Direct evidence of aspiration can also be assessed. Induced sputum can be tested for the presence of pepsin or bile acids. Bronchoalveolar lavage fluid can be examined for pepsin, bile acids, or lipid-laden macrophages.[49,50] Exhaled breath condensate pH is not specific for GER and may also be an index of airway inflammation.[51,52] More research is needed for exhaled breath condensate pH testing. Radionucleotide scanning can also show evidence of lung aspiration; however, this test is not sensitive. High-resolution computed tomography of the lung can assess end organ damage from aspiration.

Treatment

Treatment of GER-related aspiration is similar to that of GER-related asthma and chronic cough. However, speech pathologists can also provide therapy that improves upper airway protective mechanisms and swallowing function. Furthermore, substances that decrease muscle tone or arousal, including alcohol, benzodiazepines, and opiates, should be avoided. During sleep, head of bed elevation and the use of nasal continuous positive airway pressure, especially in patients with obstructive sleep apnea, decreases GER.[53]

ASPIRATION IN SPECIFIC LUNG DISEASES

Chronic Obstructive Pulmonary Disease

The role of GER in COPD is an area of increasing interest. Small studies note a relationship between GER and COPD. In a study of 42 males with severe COPD, 62% had pathologic GER by 24-hour esophageal pH monitoring, while only 42% reported GER symptoms.[54] COPD patients with GER symptoms have an increased number of COPD exacerbations (3.2/year versus 1.6/year, p = 0.02) compared to COPD patients without GER symptoms, thereby implying a causative role for GER.[55] COPD patients are also more likely to have abnormal swallowing patterns, thus increasing the risk of aspiration. This increased risk of aspiration could explain the increased rate of COPD exacerbation.[56] Terada et al examined swallowing reflexes in 67 stable COPD patients and prospectively monitored COPD exacerbations over a 12-month period. COPD patients with abnormal swallowing reflexes had more COPD exacerbations than those with normal swallowing reflexes (2.81 versus 1.56, p = 0.007). Multiple logistic regression analysis showed that abnormal swallowing reflexes were associated with 3 or more COPD exacerbations per year (odds ratio 4.86; 95% CI 1.45 to 10.43, p = 0.01).[57] One single-blinded study evaluated COPD exacerbation frequency utilizing lansoprazole 15 mg daily for 12 months in 100 COPD patients without GER symptoms. COPD exacerbation frequency was lower in the treatment group with an adjusted odds ratio, compared with the control group, of 0.23 (p = 0.004).[58] Although more research needs to be done in this area, swallowing abnormalities are common in COPD patients, and GER symptoms and swallowing abnormalities are associated with a higher frequency of COPD exacerbations.

Idiopathic Pulmonary Fibrosis and Systemic Sclerosis

Idiopathic pulmonary fibrosis (IPF) is a progressive, fibrotic pulmonary disease without a clear cause or treatment. Potentially, GER and aspiration could trigger this fibrotic response, and GER has been listed as a risk factor for IPF.[59,60] In a 2006 study, 87% of enrolled IPF patients had abnormal esophageal acid contact times, while only 47% of them had GER symptoms. Also, only 37% of the IPF patients on omeprazole 20 to 40 mg daily had normal esophageal acid contact times.[59] A case series of 4 IPF patients with GER reported stabilization or improvement of PEF with appropriate acid suppression (by PPIs or fundoplication).[60] Prospective studies are needed.

Pulmonary fibrosis is a common manifestation of systemic sclerosis, a connective tissue disease best known for its skin manifestations. Patients with systemic sclerosis frequently have severe esophageal dysfunction and GER. In a study of 40 systemic sclerosis patients, those with pulmonary fibrosis had statistically more acid and nonacid GER.[61] Investigation into the role of acid suppression and other GER therapies is needed to better determine the role aspiration plays in pulmonary fibrosis associated with systemic sclerosis.

Cystic Fibrosis

Cystic fibrosis patients have a high prevalence of GER (35% to 85%), yet 57% of cystic fibrosis patients lack typical GER symptoms.[62-64] Aspiration is associated with cystic fibrosis exacerbations. In cystic fibrosis patients treated with PPIs, 50% continue to have bile acids in their saliva.[65] Fundoplication has been shown to reduce the number of exacerbations. This suggests that nonacid reflux and aspiration may also play a role in the progression of cystic fibrosis.[65]

Lung Transplant Recipients

Aspiration may play a pivotal role in lung transplantation outcomes too. Despite the great advances in solid organ transplant in the past few decades, lung transplant recipients still face a 50%, 5-year mortality rate.[66] Much of this mortality is attributed to BOS, the equivalent of chronic rejection. BOS is an inflammatory reaction driven by multiple factors; GER and aspiration have been implicated. Median survival after BOS onset is only 3 to 4 years, so it is an area of great research interest.[66] Lung transplant recipients have many risk factors for aspiration, including vagal nerve injury during surgery, chest wall and diaphragm deformity, delayed gastric emptying due to immunosuppressive medications, impaired cilia function, and decreased cough reflex. Bile acids and pepsin are found in the bronchoalveolar lavage fluid of transplant recipients, and the presence of bile acids in the bronchoalveolar lavage fluid correlated with the presence of other inflammatory markers.[50,66] Fundoplication within 90 days of transplantation decreased the rate of BOS development.[49] Future research will assess whether treatment of nonacid GER and aspiration leads to lower rates of BOS development.

Bottom Line

GER and aspiration can affect the clinical course of many pulmonary diseases. Physicians need to be vigilant in questioning patients regarding signs and symptoms of GER and aspiration. Swallowing function testing should also be considered. Although there are no clear outcomes data, an empiric trial of PPIs may be appropriate in patients who have lung disease and GER symptoms. Fundoplication is indicated in selected patients. Attention to methods that decrease aspiration risk are also very important.

CONCLUSION AND FUTURE DIRECTIONS

GER is associated with many pulmonary diseases. Some of this is due to the organs' common embryonic origin, and some may be due to proximity in and of itself. While the advent of the PPIs has significantly improved our ability to treat acid GER, their role in the long-term management of the pulmonary manifestations of GER remains to be seen. Current recommendations suggest the use of GER lifestyle therapy and PPIs to treat patients with asthma and GER symptoms for a period of 3 months while evaluating improvement in asthma control. An empiric trial of GER lifestyle therapy and PPIs in patients with chronic cough who fit the appropriate clinical profile are recommended. Further randomized, controlled studies are needed to determine the efficacy of empiric trials in these settings. Trials investigating appropriate dose and length of GER medical therapy in these clinical settings are also needed. Medications targeting esophageal motility and transient lower esophageal sphincter relaxations are also needed to better treat GER. Lastly, we need head-to-head trials comparing the outcomes and cost benefits of medical therapy versus surgical therapy of GER in patients with lung disease.

REFERENCES

1. Maimonides M. Treatise on asthma. In: Munter S, ed. *Medical Writings of Moses Maimonides.* Philadelphia, PA: Lippincott Williams & Wilkins; 1963.
2. Harding SM. Gastroesophageal reflux: a potential asthma trigger. *Immunol Allergy Clin N Am.* 2005;25(1):131-148.
3. Mansfield LE, Hameister HH, Spaulding HS, Smith NJ, Glab N. The role of the vagus nerve in airway narrowing caused by intraesophageal hydrochloric acid provocation and esophageal distention. *Ann Allergy.* 1981;47(6):431-434.

4. Harding SM, Schan CA, Guzzo MR, Alexander RW, Bradley LA, Richter JE. Gastroesophageal reflux-induced bronchoconstriction: is microaspiration a factor? *Chest.* 1995;108(5):1220-1227.
5. Moffatt JD, Dumsday B, McLean JR, McLean JR. Non-adrenergic, non-cholinergic neurons innervating the guinea-pig trachea are located in the oesophagus: evidence from retrograde neuronal tracing. *Neurosci Lett.* 1998;248(1):37-40.
6. Herve P, Denjean A, Jian R, Simmonneau G, Duroux P. Intraesophageal perfusion of acid increases the bronchomotor response to methacholine and to isocapnic hyperventilation in asthmatic subjects. *Am Rev Respir Dis.* 1986;134(5):986-989.
7. Jack CI, Calverley PM, Donnelly RJ, et al. Simultaneous tracheal and oesophageal pH measurements in asthmatic patients with gastro-oesophageal pH measurements in asthmatic patients with gastro-oesophageal reflux. *Thorax.* 1995;50(2):201-204.
8. Tuchman DN, Boyle JT, Pack AI, et al. Comparison of airway responses following tracheal or esophageal acidification in the cat. *Gastroenterology.* 1984;87(4):872-881.
9. Hamamoto J, Kohrogi H, Kawano O, et al. Esophageal stimulation by hydrochloric acid causes neurogenic inflammation in airways in guinea pigs. *J Appl Physiol.* 1997;82(3):738-745.
10. Zerbib F, Guisset O, Lamouliatte H, Quinton JP, Galmiche JP, Tunon-De-Lara JM. Effects of bronchial obstruction on lower esophageal sphincter motility and gastroesophageal reflux in patients with asthma. *Am J Respir Crit Care Med.* 2002;166(9):1206-1211.
11. Sontag SJ, O'Connell S, Khandelwal S, et al. Most asthmatics have gastroesophageal reflux with or without bronchodilator therapy. *Gastroenterology.* 1990;99(3):613-620.
12. Ruigómez A, Rodriguez LA, Wallander MA, Johansson S, Thomas M, Price D. Gastroesophageal reflux disease and asthma. *Chest.* 2005;128(1):85-93.
13. El-Serag HB, Sonnenberg A. Comorbid occurrence of laryngeal or pulmonary disease with esophagitis in United States military veterans. *Gastroenterology.* 1997;113(3):755-760.
14. Sontag SJ, Schnell TG, Miller TQ, et al. Prevalence of oesophagitis in asthmatics. *Gut.* 1992;33(7):872-876.
15. Field SK, Underwood M, Brant R, Cowie RL. Prevalence of gastroesophageal reflux symptoms in asthma. *Chest.* 1996;109(2):316-322.
16. Harding SM, Guzzo MR, Richter JE. 24-h esophageal pH testing in asthmatics. *Chest.* 1999;115(3):654-659.
17. Harding SM, Guzzo MR, Richter JE. The prevalence of gastroesophageal reflux in asthma patients without reflux symptoms. *Am J Respir Crit Care Med.* 2000;162(1):34-39.
18. Lazenby JP, Guzzo MR, Harding SM, Patterson PE, Johnson LF, Bradley LA. Oral corticosteroids increase esophageal acid contact times in patients with stable asthma. *Chest.* 2002;121(2):625-634.
19. Harding SM, Richter JE, Guzzo MR, Schan CA, Alexander RW, Bradley LA. Asthma and gastroesophageal reflux: acid suppressive therapy improves asthma outcome. *Am J Med.* 1996;100(4):395-405.
20. DiMango E, Holbrook JT, Simpson E, et al. Effects of asymptomatic proximal and distal gastroesophageal reflux on asthma severity. *Am J Respir Crit Care Med.* 2009;180(9):809-816.
21. National Asthma Education and Prevention Program. Expert Panel Report 3 (EPR-3). Guidelines for the diagnosis and management of asthma. Summary report 2007. *J Allergy Clin Immunol.* 2007;120 (5 suppl):S94-S138.
22. Gibson PG, Henry RL, Coughlan JL. Gastro-oesophageal reflux treatment for asthma in adults and children. *Cochrane Database Syst Rev.* 2003;(2):CD001496.
23. American Lung Association Asthma Clinical Research Centers; Mastronarde JG, Anthonisen NR, Castro M, et al. Efficacy of esomeprazole for treatment of poorly controlled asthma. *N Engl J Med.* 2009;360(15):1487-1499.
24. Littner MR, Leung FX, Ballard ED, Huang B, Samra NK; Lansoprazole Asthma Study Group. Effects of 24 weeks of lansoprazole therapy on asthma symptoms, exacerbations, quality of life, and pulmonary function in adult asthmatic patients with acid reflux symptoms. *Chest.* 2005;128(3):1128-1135.
25. Kiljander TO, Harding SM, Field SK, et al. Effects of esomeprazole 40 mg twice daily on asthma: a randomized placebo-controlled trial. *Am J Respir Crit Care Med.* 2006;173(10):1091-1097.
26. Kiljander TO, Junghard O, Beckman O, Lind T. Effect of esomeprazole 40 mg once or twice daily on asthma: a randomized, placebo-controlled study. *Am J Respir Crit Care Med.* 2010;181(10):1042-1048.
27. Field SK, Gelfand GA, McFadden SD. The effects of antireflux surgery on asthmatics with gastroesophageal reflux. *Chest.* 1999;116(3):766-774.
28. Larrain A, Carrasco E, Galleguillos F, Sepulveda R, Pope CE 2nd. Medical and surgical treatment of nonallergic asthma associated with gastroesophageal reflux. *Chest.* 1991;99(6):1330-1335.
29. Sontag SJ, O'Connell S, Khandelwal S, et al. Asthmatics with gastroesophageal reflux: long term results of a randomized trial of medical and surgical antireflux therapies. *Am J Gastroenterol.* 2003;98(5):987-999.
30. Irwin RS. Chronic cough due to gastroesophageal reflux disease: ACCP evidence-based clinical practice guidelines. *Chest.* 2006;129(1 suppl):80S-94S.

31. Irwin RS, Boulet LP, Cloutier MM, et al. Managing cough as a defense mechanism and as a symptom. A consensus panel report of the American College of Chest Physicians. *Chest.* 1998;114(2 suppl):133S-181S.

32. Chandra KM, Harding SM. Therapy insight: treatment of gastroesophageal reflux in adults with chronic cough. *Nat Clin Pract Gastroenterol Hepatol.* 2007;4(11):604-613.

33. Pratter MR. Overview of common causes of cough: ACCP evidence-based clinical practice guidelines. *Chest.* 2006;129(1 suppl):59S-62S.

34. Sifrim D, Dupont L, Blondeau K, Zhang X, Janssens J. Weakly acidic reflux in patients with chronic unexplained cough during 24 hour pressure, pH, and impedance monitoring. *Gut.* 2005;54(4):449-454.

35. Irwin RS, French CL, Curley FJ, Zawacki JK, Bennett FM. Chronic cough due to gastroesophageal reflux: clinical, diagnostic, and pathogenetic aspects. *Chest.* 1993;104(5):1511-1517.

36. Morice AH, McGarvey L, Pavord I; British Thoracic Society Cough Guideline Group. Recommendations for the management of cough in adults. *Thorax.* 2006;61(suppl 1):11-24.

37. Poe RH, Kallay MC. Chronic cough and gastroesophageal reflux disease: experience with specific therapy for diagnosis and treatment. *Chest.* 2003;123(3):679-684.

38. Patterson N, Mainie I, Rafferty G, et al. Nonacid reflux episodes reaching the pharynx are important factors associated with cough. *J Clin Gastroenterol.* 2009;43(5):414-419.

39. Vaezi MF, Richter JE. Twenty-four-hour ambulatory esophageal pH monitoring in the diagnosis of acid reflux-related chronic cough. *South Med J.* 1997;90(3):305-311.

40. Ours TM, Kavuru MS, Schilz RJ, Richter JE. A prospective evaluation of esophageal testing and a double-blind, randomized study of omeprazole in a diagnostic and therapeutic algorithm for chronic cough. *Am J Gastroenterol.* 1999;94(11):3131-3138.

41. Irwin RS, Curley FJ, French CL. Chronic cough. The spectrum and frequency of causes, key components of the diagnostic evaluation, and outcome of specific therapy. *Am Rev Respir Dis.* 1990;141(3):640-647.

42. Esomeprazole (Nexium). *Physicians' Desk Reference 2009.* 63rd ed. Montvale, NJ: Thomson Reuters; 645-654.

43. Chang AB, Lasserson TJ, Gaffney J, Connor FL, Garske LA. Gastro-oesophageal reflux treatment for prolonged non-specific cough in children and adults. *Cochrane Database Syst Rev.* 2006;(4):CD004823.

44. Kiljander TO, Salomaa ER, Hietanen EK, Terho EO. Chronic cough and gastro-oesophageal reflux: a double-blind placebo-controlled study with omeprazole. *Eur Respir J.* 2000;16(4):633-638.

45. Mainie I, Tutuian R, Agrawal A, et al. Fundoplication eliminates chronic cough due to non-acid reflux identified by impedance pH monitoring. *Thorax.* 2005;60(6):521-523.

46. Allen CJ, Anvari M. Does laparoscopic fundoplication provide long-term control of gastroesophageal reflux-related cough? *Surg Endosc.* 2004;18(4):633-637.

47. Liu JJ, Carr-Locke DL, Osterman MT, et al. Endoscopic treatment for atypical manifestations of gastro-esophageal reflux disease. *Am J Gastroenterol.* 2006;101(3):440-445.

48. Effros RM, Jacobs ER, Schapira RM, Biller J. Response of the lungs to aspiration. *Am J Med.* 2000;108(suppl 4a):15S-19S.

49. Cantu E 3rd, Appel JZ 3rd, Hartwig G, et al. J Maxwell Chamberlain memorial paper. Early fundoplication prevents chronic allograft dysfunction in patients with gastroesophageal reflux disease. *Ann Thorac Surg.* 2004;78(4):1142-1151.

50. D'Ovidio F, Mura M, Tsang M, et al. Bile acid aspiration and the development of bronchiolitis obliterans after lung transplantation. *J Thorac Cardiovasc Surg.* 2005;129(5):1144-1152.

51. Effros RM, Su J, Casaburi R, Shaker R, Biller J, Dunning M. Utility of exhaled breath condensates in chronic obstructive pulmonary disease: a critical review. *Curr Opin Pulm Med.* 2005;11(2):135-139.

52. Davis CS, Gagermeier J, Dilling D, et al. A review of the potential applications and controversies of non-invasive testing for biomarkers of aspiration in the lung transplant population. *Clin Transplant.* 2010;24(3):E54-E61.

53. Tawk M, Goodrich S, Kinasewitz G, Orr W. The effect of 1 week of continuous positive airway pressure treatment in obstructive sleep apnea patients with concomitant gastroesophageal reflux. *Chest.* 2006;130(4):1003-1008.

54. Casanova C, Baudet JS, del Valle Velasco M, et al. Increased gastro-oesophageal reflux disease in patients with severe COPD. *Eur Respir J.* 2004;23(6):841-845.

55. Rascon-Aguilar IE, Pamer M, Wludyka P, et al. Role of gastroesophageal reflux symptoms in exacerbations of COPD. *Chest.* 2006;130(4):1096-1101.

56. Gross RD, Atwood CW Jr, Ross SB, Olszewski JW, Eichhorn KA. The coordination of breathing and swallowing in chronic obstructive pulmonary disease. *Am J Respir Crit Care Med.* 2009;179(7):559-565.

57. Terada K, Muro S, Ohara T, et al. Abnormal swallowing reflex and COPD exacerbations. *Chest.* 2010;137(2):326-332.

58. Sasaki T, Nakayama K, Yasuda H, et al. A randomized, single-blind study of lansoprazole for the prevention of exacerbations of chronic obstructive pulmonary disease in older patients. *J Am Geriatr Soc.* 2009;57(8):1453-1457.

59. Raghu G, Freudenberger TD, Yang S, et al. High prevalence of abnormal acid gastro-oesophageal reflux in idiopathic pulmonary fibrosis. *Eur Respir J.* 2008;27(1);136-142.
60. Raghu G, Yang S, Spada C, Hayes J, Pellegrini CA. Sole treatment of acid gastroesophageal reflux in idiopathic pulmonary fibrosis: a case series. *Chest.* 2006;19(3):794-800.
61. Savarino E, Bazzica M, Zentilin P, et al. Gastroesophageal reflux and pulmonary fibrosis in scleroderma. A study using pH-impedance monitoring. *Am J Respir Crit Care Med.* 2009;179(5):408-413.
62. Button BM, Roberts S, Kotsimbos TC, et al. Gastroesophageal reflux (symptomatic and silent): a potentially significant problem in patients with cystic fibrosis before and after lung transplantation. *J Heart Lung Transplant.* 2005;24(10):1522-1529.
63. Blondeau K, DuPont LJ, Mertens V, et al. Gastro-oesophageal reflux and aspiration of gastric contents in adult patients with cystic fibrosis. *Gut.* 2008;57(8):1049-1055.
64. Sabati AA, Kempainen RR, Milla CE, et al. Characteristics of gastroesophageal reflux in adults with cystic fibrosis. *J Cyst Fibros.* 2010;9(5):365-370.
65. Fathi H, Moon T, Donaldson J, Jackson W, Sedman P, Morice AH. Cough in adult cystic fibrosis: diagnosis and response to fundoplication. *Cough.* 2009;5:1.
66. Blondeau K, Mertens V, Vanaudenaerde BA et al. Gastro-oesophageal reflux and gastric aspiration in lung transplant patients with or without chronic rejection. *Eur Respir J.* 2008;31(4):707-713.

Ear, Nose, and Throat Manifestations of GERD

An Otolaryngologist's Perspective

Joseph R. Spiegel, MD

Laryngopharyngeal reflux (LPR) is the term used for the effects of reflux of stomach contents on the structures of the upper aerodigestive tract. The diagnosis and treatment of LPR has had a significant impact on the practice of otolaryngology. From 1990 to 1993, annual visits to otolaryngologists for reflux-related problems averaged 89,000/year and by 1998 to 2001 increased to 421,000/year. However, the diagnosis and treatment of LPR remains controversial. The signs and symptoms of LPR are nonspecific, and there remains a lack of large, well-controlled studies to document its response to treatment.

CHRONIC LARYNGITIS

The laryngeal mucosa is thin, and there are dense sensory nerve connections in the larynx and pharynx, unlike in the lower esophagus. Acute and chronic symptoms of irritation can result from mild inflammatory changes. Koufman[1] found laryngeal inflammation after as few as 3 exposures (pH < 4) per week. Studies of pH probe findings in patients with presumed LPR show a wide range in the pattern of proximal acid exposure and little correlation to the frequency of exposure and the intensity of symptoms.[2] More recently, the presence of pepsin in pharyngeal refluxate has been implicated as a possible cofactor in laryngeal mucosal inflammation.[3]

The most common symptoms ascribed to LPR are frequent throat clearing, globus, cough, hoarseness, choking episodes, and dysphagia. Globus is best described as a foreign

DiMarino AJ Jr, Cohen S, eds.
Extraesophageal Manifestations of GERD (pp 51-72).
© 2013 Taylor & Francis Group.

body sensation in the throat, and it is separate from dysphagia. Many patients with globus will describe improvement when they swallow food or liquids. Dysphagia can be associated with LPR, especially when there is a component of cricopharyngeal dysfunction. However, patients with dysphagia caused by reflux-related mid and lower esophageal pathology can often present with symptoms of choking and cervical-level dysphagia, placing both gastroesophageal reflux disease (GERD) and LPR in the differential diagnosis. Hoarseness has multiple etiologies, and many patients with hoarseness complaints have multifactorial causation. Even patients found to have a vocal cord malignancy as a cause of their voice change often have a long history of hoarseness related to common cofactors of smoking, reflux, dehydration, and voice abuse. Patients with dysphagia and/ or hoarseness will often be diagnosed with LPR. However, it may be difficult to determine the role of laryngeal reflux in the development of these multifactorial symptoms.

A careful history is necessary to assess other potential causes for these symptoms (eg, allergies, chronic rhinosinusitis [CRS], tobacco use, alcohol use, and the side effects of certain drugs). Most patients with laryngeal complaints of reflux do not have classic symptoms of heartburn.[4]

Otolaryngologists depend on laryngoscopy as the initial diagnostic test. This can be performed with a mirror but is most often performed as transnasal fiber optic endoscopy. It also can be performed with a transoral rigid telescope. The most common signs ascribed to LPR are erythema and edema of the posterior mucosa, irregularity of the intra-arytenoid mucosa, hyperplasia of the postcricoid mucosa, obliteration of the laryngeal ventricle, and pseudosulcus.[5] Examples of these changes can be seen in Figure 4-1. It is difficult to depend solely on these physical findings for the diagnosis of LPR because of the presence of these signs in "normal" patients[6] and the inability to establish repeatable grading of laryngeal exams with multiple evaluators.[7] A reflux finding score based on 8 laryngeal findings has been proposed by Belafsky et al.[8] It has been validated with small study groups, but it is not widely used in practice.

Hoarseness may result directly from mucosal inflammation or from the more chronic effect of repeated irritation on laryngeal motion. Both vocal fold and subglottic edema have been reported as signs of LPR. Additionally, chronic edema in the posterior laryngeal tissues can impede normal laryngeal closure. All of these changes can lead to a pattern of compensatory hyperfunction (ie, muscle tension dysphonia) that compounds the voice change resulting from inflammation alone.[9] Control of LPR is considered an adjunct to voice therapy in the treatment of muscle tension dysphonia. Patients with cough and asthma often benefit from reflux treatment.[10] Both cough and asthma can contribute to hoarseness through chronic laryngeal trauma and loss of breath support for speaking. Thus, when treatment for reflux helps control these complaints, it can also indirectly be a part of treatment for hoarseness as well.

Treatment of chronic laryngeal symptoms attributed to LPR is based on a treatment trial of proton pump inhibitors (PPIs), diet changes, and behavioral modification. Trials of 2 to 4 months have been suggested. A meta-analysis of randomized, controlled studies of PPI treatment in suspected LPR showed mixed responses and no overall significant difference between responses to PPIs or placebos.[11] When a patient is placed on a treatment trial for chronic laryngeal symptoms, it is important to define the symptoms being monitored and to document adherence to treatment. When laryngeal symptoms resolve during treatment, trials of reduction or cessation of PPI treatment can be helpful in establishing the benefit of long-term PPI treatment.

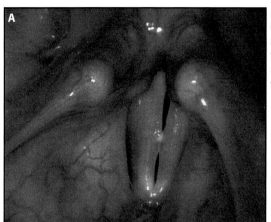

Figure 4-1. Findings of LPR on laryngoscopy. (A) Hyperemia and erythema over the arytenoid mucosa. (B) Discolored hypertrophic intra-arytenoid tissue. (C) Severe mucosal erythema and edema of the posterior larynx.

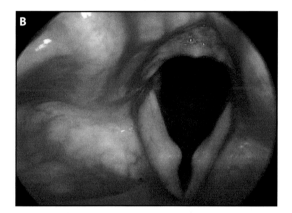

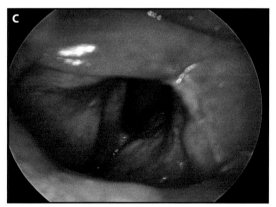

LARYNGEAL CANCER

GERD has been implicated as a possible etiological factor in the causation of laryngeal cancer. Laryngeal cancer has an annual incidence in the United States of 11,300 and a mortality of 3600.[12] Case-control studies have shown an increased risk of laryngeal cancer in patients with a history of GERD symptoms.[13-15] Specifically, GERD has been implicated as increasing the risk of laryngeal cancer in active cigarette smokers. Other studies have not shown evidence of an association.[16,17] The difficulty in retrospective analysis lies in the accurate diagnosis of GERD and the similarity of LPR symptoms to those of early laryngeal cancer. Although the evidence is not clear enough to consider GERD a primary etiological factor in laryngeal cancer, control of reflux is considered important in patients with premalignant changes in the larynx and those undergoing treatment for laryngeal malignancy.

CHRONIC RHINOSINUSITIS

CRS is a multifactorial disease that results from mucosal inflammation leading to sinus obstruction, mucosal stasis, and subsequent infection. Allergies and anatomic abnormalities are predisposing factors, and infections may be viral, bacterial, or fungal.[18] Extraesophageal reflux has been implicated as a possible additional cause of mucosal inflammation leading to the cascade of CRS.[19] Nasopharyngeal exposure to reflux has been found in pH probes in both children and adults.[20,21] Other studies have shown the presence of gastric pepsin in sinus tissue, nasopharyngeal secretions, and middle ear effusions.[22,23] In clinical studies, the initiation of treatment for reflux in patients with symptoms of CRS has resulted in symptom improvement.[24] In clinical practice, treatment for reflux should be considered in pediatric patients with chronic sinusitis and in adults with symptoms of CRS that have not responded to more traditional regimens.

OTITIS MEDIA

Extraesophageal reflux has been implicated as an etiological factor in otitis media with effusion, especially in infants. Both conditions are very common in the first year of life. Animal studies have shown that acid exposure in the nasopharynx can lead to transient eustachian tube dysfunction.[25] More recent studies have shown the presence of pepsin/pepsinogen in the middle ear cleft with a much higher prevalence in children with purulent otitis media than in the control group.[26] However, a clinical history of GERD, allergy, or asthma did not correlate with findings of extraesophageal reflux in the middle ear.

SUBGLOTTIC STENOSIS

The development of subglottic stenosis is most often multifactorial. In neonates and infants, congenital stenosis must be considered. Many infants have frequent reflux of gastric contents, and if these children require intubation for any reason, reflux has been implicated as a factor in the subsequent development of laryngeal or tracheal stenosis.[27] However, in this population, control of reflux is not controversial as it is a necessary component of their care to establish a normal pattern of oral feeding in addition to reducing the risk of airway complications.

In adults, LPR has been considered as a probable etiological factor in patients defined as having idiopathic subglottic stenosis. These patients have no risk factors of inflammatory diseases, such as Wegner's granulomatosis or sarcoidosis, and no history of laryngeal trauma or endotracheal intubation. Maronian et al found a strong association of positive pH probe studies (pharyngeal pH < 4) in this group, but only 7 patients were available for evaluation.[28] There is also an overwhelming female predominance in patients with idiopathic subglottic stenosis. Damrose recently published a hypothesis for the development of this condition due to anatomic and hormonal factors alone.[29]

ONGOING CONTROVERSIES

Otolaryngologists consider LPR a primary cause of common symptoms of laryngeal and throat irritation and a secondary cause of more distant chronic inflammation in the nose, paranasal sinuses, and middle ear. The symptoms of LPR represent common irritative complaints that can be caused by multiple etiologies, both chronic and acute. Studies published in otolaryngological literature have thus far utilized relatively small numbers of patients and have failed to establish distinct diagnostic criteria for LPR or endpoints for treatment. The most comprehensive recent reviews suggest provisional diagnosis based primarily on symptoms and secondarily on physical findings, with confirmation by a 3- to 4-month trial of medical and behavioral control of reflux. There are ongoing investigations regarding patients who continue to have symptoms at the laryngeal level despite an adequate trial of medical treatment and behavioral controls. A recent study of patients with chronic cough who had been unresponsive to treatment for the most common causes (including reflux) showed as much as a 75% long-term response rate to treatment for vagal neuropathy.[30] Control of this factor may help determine the true role of reflux as a cough trigger.

Salminen et al have shown a reduction in laryngeal symptoms in patients who underwent Nissen fundoplication for GERD.[31] However, other studies have failed to show a consistent relief of laryngeal symptoms after fundoplication in those patients who noted relief of GERD symptoms.[32,33] At this time, Nissen fundoplication cannot be relied upon to provide consistent treatment of extraesophageal reflux symptoms. In the absence of surgical indications for GERD, there are no reliable indications to suggest fundoplication in the treatment of extraesophageal reflux symptoms alone. There are also many studies on the role of laryngeal exposure to pepsin, even in patients with adequate gastric acid control.[22,34] This may lead to new methods of detecting refluxate at the laryngeal and pharyngeal level, and perhaps result in new stratagems of treatment to reduce the effects of pepsin exposure.

The basic guidelines for evaluation and treatment of LPR have been developed but remain rudimentary due to a lack of definitive diagnostic criteria and endpoints of treatment. The association of LPR with GERD, and the attendant cancer risk of Barrett's esophagus, remains unclear. The risk of LPR as a contributing factor in laryngeal cancer is suspected but not firmly established. Further study will allow firmer guidelines that will allow for adequate surveillance for patients at risk and appropriate utilization of medical resources for symptomatic patients.

REFERENCES

1. Koufman JA. The otolaryngologic manifestations of gastroesophageal reflux disease (GERD): a clinical investigation of 225 patients using ambulatory 24-hour pH monitoring and an experimental investigation of the role of acid and pepsin in the development of laryngeal injury. *Laryngoscope.* 1991;101(4 pt 2 suppl 53):1–78.
2. Noordzij JP, Khidr A, Desper E, Meek RB, Feibel JF, Levine PA. Correlation of pH probe-measured laryngopharyngeal reflux with symptoms and signs of reflux laryngitis. *Laryngoscope.* 2002;112:2192-2195.
3. Johnston N, Knight J, Dettmar PW, Lively MO, Koufman J. Pepsin and carbonic anhydrase isoenzyme III as diagnostic markers for laryngopharyngeal reflux disease. *Laryngoscope.* 2004;114:2129-2134.
4. Koufman JA. Laryngopharyngeal reflux is different from classic gastroesophageal reflux disease. *Ear Nose Throat J.* 2002;81(suppl 2):7-9.
5. Vaezi MF, Hicks DM, Abelson TI, Richter JE. Laryngeal signs and symptoms and gastroesophageal reflux disease (GERD): a critical assessment of cause and effect association. *Clin Gastroenterol Hepatol.* 2003;1:333-344.

6. Milstein CF, Charbel S, Hicks DM, Abelson TI, Richter JE, Vaezi MF. Prevalence of laryngeal irritation signs associated with reflux in asymptomatic volunteers: impact of endoscopic technique (rigid vs flexible scope). *Laryngoscope.* 2005;115:2256-2261.

7. Branski RC, Bhattacharyya N, Shapiro J. The reliability of the assessment of endoscopic laryngeal findings associated with laryngopharyngeal reflux disease. *Laryngoscope.* 2002;112:1019-1024.

8. Belafsky PC, Postma GN, Koufman JA. The validity and reliability of the reflux finding score (RFS). *Laryngoscope.* 2001;111:1313-1317.

9. Cesari U, Galli J, Ricciardiello F, Cavaliere M, Galli V. Dysphonia and laryngopharyngeal reflux. *Acta Otorhinolaryngologica Italica.* 2004;24(1):13-19.

10. Chandra KM, Harding SM, Therapy insight: treatment of gastroesophageal reflux in adults with chronic cough. *Nat Clin Pract Gastroenterol Hepatol.* 2007;4(11):604-613.

11. Qadeer MA, Phillips CO, Lopez AR, et al. Proton pump inhibitor therapy for suspected GERD-related chronic laryngitis: a meta analysis of randomized controlled trials. *Am J Gastroenterol.* 2006;101:2646-2654.

12. Chu EA, Kim YJ. Laryngeal cancer: diagnosis and preoperative work-up. *Otolaryngol Clin North Am.* 2008;41:673-695.

13. Qadeer MA, Cammarota N, Vaezi MF. Is GERD a risk factor for laryngeal cancer? *Laryngoscope.* 2005;115:486-491.

14. Lewis JS, Gillenwater AM, Garrett JD, et al. Characterization of laryngopharyngeal reflux in patients with premalignant or early carcinomas of the larynx. *Cancer.* 2003;97:1010-1014.

15. Vaezi MF, Qadeer MA, Lopez R, Colabianchi N. Laryngeal cancer and gastroesophageal reflux disease: a case-control study. *Am J Med.* 2006;119:768-776.

16. Wilson JA. What is the evidence that gastroesophageal reflux is involved in the etiology of laryngeal cancer? *Curr Opin Otolaryngolol Head Neck Surg.* 2005;13:97-100.

17. Ozlugedik S, Yorulmaz J, Gokcan K. Is laryngopharyngeal reflux an important risk factor in the development of laryngeal carcinoma? *Eur Arch Otorhinolaryngol.* 2006;263:339-343.

18. Kennedy DW. Pathogenesis of chronic rhinosinusitis. *Ann Otol Rhinol Laryngol.* 2004;193(suppl):6-9.

19. Loehrl TA, Smith TL, Darling RJ. Autonomic dysfunction, vasomotor rhinitis and extraesophageal reflux. *Otolaryngol Head Neck Surg.* 2002;126:382-387.

20. Contencin P, Narcy P. Nasopharyngeal pH monitoring in infants and children with chronic rhinopharyngitis. *Int J Ped Otorhinolaryngol.* 1991;22:249-256.

21. DelGaudio JM. Direct nasopharyngeal reflux of gastric acid is a contributing factor in refractory chronic rhinosinusitis. *Laryngoscope.* 2005;115:946-957.

22. Ozmen S, Yucel OT, Sinici I, et al. Nasal pepsin assay and pH monitoring in chronic rhinosinusitis. *Laryngoscope.* 2008;118:890-894.

23. Tasker A, Dettmar PW, Panetti M, Kaufmann JA. Is gastric reflux a cause of otitis media with effusion in children. *Laryngoscope.* 2002;112:1930-1934.

24. Bothwell MR, Parson DS, Talbot A. Outcome of reflux therapy on pediatric chronic sinusitis. *Otolaryngol Head Neck Surg.* 1999;121:255-262.

25. Heavner SB, Hardy SM, White DR, Prazma J, Pillsbury HC. Transient inflammation and dysfunction of the eustachian tube secondary to multiple exposures of simulated gastroesophageal refluxant. *Ann Otol Rhinol Laryngol.* 2001;110:928-934.

26. O'Reilly RC, Zhaoping H, Bloedon E, et al. The role of extraesophageal reflux in otitis media in infants and children. *Laryngoscope.* 2008;118(suppl):1-9.

27. Halstead LA. Gastroesophageal reflux: a critical factor in pediatric subglottic stenosis. *Otolaryng Head Neck Surg.* 1999;120:683-688.

28. Maronian NC, Asadeh H, Waugh P, Hillel A. Association of laryngopharyngeal reflux disease and subglottic stenosis. *Ann Oto Rhin Laryng.* 2001;110:606-612.

29. Damrose EJ. On the development of idiopathic subglottic stenosis. *Med Hypotheses.* 2008;71:122-125.

30. Spiegel JR. Neuropathic cough: outcomes of medical treatment in 138 cases. Submitted for publication, February 2012.

31. Salminen P, Karvonen J, Ovaska J. Long-term outcomes after laparascopic Nissen fundoplication for reflux laryngitis. *Dig Surg.* 2010;27(6):509-514.

32. So JB, Zeitels SM, Rattner DW. Outcomes of atypical symptoms attributed to gastroesophageal reflux treated by laparoscopic fundoplication. *Surgery.* 1998;124(1):28-32.

33. Swoger J, Ponsky J, Hicks DM, et al. Surgical fundoplication in laryngopharyngeal reflux unresponsive to aggressive acid suppression: a controlled study. *Clin Gastroenterol Hepatol.* 2006;4(4):433-441.

34. Bulmer DM, Ali MS, Brownlee IA, Dettmar PW, Pearson JP, Laryngeal mucosa: its susceptibility to damage by acid and pepsin. *Laryngoscope.* 2008;120:777-782.

Table 4-1	Symptoms Attributed to Laryngopharyngeal Reflux
• Hoarseness • Dysphonia • Sore or burning throat • Excessive throat clearing • Chronic cough	• Globus pharyngeus • Dysphagia • Postnasal drip • Laryngospasm

A Gastroenterologist's Perspective

Lisa S. Cassani, MD and Michael F. Vaezi, MD, PhD, MSc

LPR, or *laryngopharyngeal reflux*, is a term commonly used by ear, nose, and throat (ENT) specialists to describe the GER, or gastroesophageal reflux, that reaches the anatomical structures above the upper esophageal sphincter (eg, the laryngeal or pharyngeal mucosa). Other commonly employed terminology include *reflux laryngitis* or *GER-related laryngitis*. As controversial as the terminology defining the disease might appear, it pales in comparison to identifying which patients actually have the disease and in whom it is overly or incorrectly diagnosed. For sake of simplicity, we will employ the term *LPR* to refer to a disease state in which patients have throat symptoms "felt to be" GER related. Presenting symptoms of suspected LPR may include chronic cough, sore throat, throat clearing, hoarseness, and globus sensation to name a few (Table 4-1). LPR is among the extraesophageal syndromes of reflux disease with varying symptom presentation, and many patients may not report the concomitant presence of the classical symptoms of reflux such as heartburn. This results in added complexity to diagnosing true GER-related findings and symptoms in patients with suspected extraesophageal reflux.[1,2] In this chapter, we will review the current understanding and dilemma in the diagnoses and management of patients with various throat symptoms and discuss their often controversial link to GER.

Two proposed mechanisms of extraesophageal symptoms include microaspiration of gastric or duodenal contents and stimulation of a vagal reflex arc. Protective structures to prevent the former are the gastrointestinal junctional structures (which include the lower and upper esophageal sphincters), peristaltic actions of the esophagus, acid neutralization by saliva, protective airway reflexes (including the esophagoglottal closure and the cough reflexes), and mucociliary clearance.[3] Potential caustic offenders include gastric acid and pepsin as well as duodenal bile acids and trypsin. Injury secondary to acid and pepsin is a well-known causative factor in esophagitis. Animal studies have also documented injurious potential in laryngeal lesions for both gastric as well as duodenal agents.[4-7] However, it appears that bile constituents such as trypsin and conjugated and unconjugated bile acids cause minimal histologic change in the absence of acid.[6] Less acidic or nonacid refluxate can, however, produce symptoms such as regurgitation, which may not be effectively treated with PPIs. The intermittent nature of some gastroduodenal reflux poses a challenge for the less than perfect diagnostic tests currently available.

As the initial test performed by our ENT colleagues in patients with chronic throat symptoms, laryngoscopy is sensitive but not specific enough to diagnose GER-related LPR.[2] It is able to identify laryngeal irritation but cannot distinguish GER-related irritants

Table 4-2	Potential Laryngopharyngeal Signs Associated With Gastroesophageal Reflux
• Edema and hyperemia of larynx • Hyperemia and lymphoid hyperplasia of posterior pharynx (cobblestoning) • Granuloma • Contact ulcers • Laryngeal polyps	• Interarytenoid changes • Reinke's edema • Tumors • Subglottic stenosis • Posterior glottic stenosis

Figure 4-2. Normal laryngeal tissue. AC indicates arytenoid complex; AMW, arytenoid medial wall; FVF, false vocal fold; PCW, posterior cricoid wall; PPW, posterior pharyngeal wall; TVF, true vocal fold.

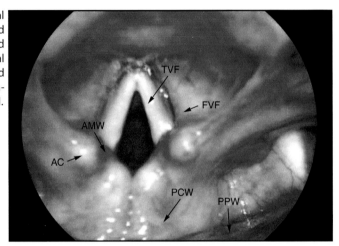

from other potential irritants. Contact ulcers in the larynx were the first laryngeal signs associated with GER.[4] Since then, additional laryngeal findings (eg, edema, erythema, and nodularity of the posterior larynx, the arytenoids, and the interarytenoid area) have also been implicated in reflux (Table 4-2 and Figures 4-2 and 4-3). However, many such laryngeal findings may be the result of irritants such as smoking and environmental allergens.[8] The subtle signs of irritation often found in GER-related LPR are commonly present in healthy volunteers.[2,9] The lack of specificity hinders the use of laryngoscopy as a means of diagnostic testing for LPR.[10] Further evidence for laryngoscopy as a poor diagnostic tool is that up to 50% of patients with laryngoscopic signs suggesting GER do not respond to aggressive acid suppression and do not have abnormal esophageal acid reflux values on pH testing. Qadeer et al reported a poor correlation between signs of laryngeal inflammation and patient symptoms in those suspected of having LPR 1-year post-Nissen fundoplication.[11] Given the poor specificity of laryngoscopy in diagnosing GER-related laryngeal changes, it is not surprising that many are incorrectly diagnosed as LPR who may not have reflux disease at all.

The diagnostic tools available to gastroenterologists are equally poor in differentiating GER-related laryngeal changes from other potential causes. In a given patient with chronic throat symptoms who is referred to a gastroenterologist, esophagogastroduodenoscopy and/or pH monitoring are often the initial diagnostic tests performed.[12] However, neither test is a gold standard in establishing a true relationship between patients' symptoms and GER. This is in part due to overdiagnosis of LPR and in part due to poor sensitivity of

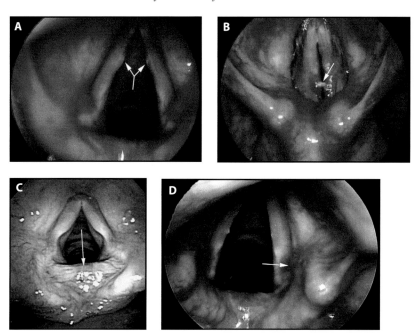

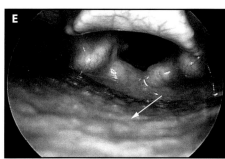

Figure 4-3. Abnormal larynx. (A) Bilateral true vocal fold nodules. (B) True vocal fold erythema. (C) Interarytenoid bar. (D) Arytenoid medial wall erythema. (E) Posterior pharyngeal wall cobblestoning.

the tests. Less than 30% of patients with extraesophageal manifestations show endoscopic evidence of esophagitis at endoscopy.[13] In one study by Baldi and colleagues, 45 patients with chronic cough were evaluated with esophagogastroduodenoscopy finding that only 15.5% of all the patients, regardless of these classic symptoms, had erosive esophagitis on endoscopy. The authors correctly concluded that "upper [gastrointestinal] endoscopy has a very low sensitivity in patients with atypical GER symptoms and, in the absence of other clinical indications, should not be included in the diagnostic work-up of these patients."[14]

Similarly, the clinical utility of prolonged esophageal or pharyngeal pH monitoring should be scrutinized. Approximately 50% to 80% of patients with suspected GER have abnormal acid exposure, irrespective of pH probe placement.[2,13,15,16] Vaezi et al studied reproducibility and reliability of the proximal pH probe in detecting proximal esophageal reflux and found excellent specificity at 91% but poorer sensitivity and reproducibility at 55%, indicating that a negative result does not rule out the possibility of proximal reflux.[17] In addition, Park et al demonstrated that pretherapy demographics, presenting symptoms, pH monitoring, and esophageal manometry were not predictive of 4-month treatment outcome in patients referred for suspected LPR.[18] There is also poor consensus on the "normal" values of proximal or hypopharyngeal pH measurements and where exactly to place the proximal probe in dual-probe monitoring.[2,7,13,19] A pH of less than 4 in the esophagus had originally been shown to have high sensitivity and specificity,[20] but recently a cutoff of a pH less than 5 has been suggested to be more specific for LPR.[21] Further trials will be needed to determine more precisely what pH threshold is necessary for the diagnosis of LPR. Hypopharyngeal pH monitoring was initially believed to be more accurate than pH monitoring in the distal or proximal esophagus for patients with LPR. Shaker et al studied 3-site pH probes in 14 patients with both laryngeal signs and symptoms, 12 patients with laryngeal symptoms only, 16 patients with esophageal reflux symptoms without laryngeal symptoms, and 12 controls. In this study, hypopharyngeal reflux was more frequent and in greater quantity in patients with laryngeal signs and symptoms.[22] However, hypopharyngeal pH monitoring has several limitations. One issue is that up to 17% of normal patients demonstrated hypopharyngeal reflux events.[23] This rate varies between 7% to 17%.[24,25] Additionally, Vaezi showed that only 54% of 1217 patients with suspected LPR had abnormal esophageal acid exposure regardless of where the pH probe was placed.[26] More importantly, Ulualp et al found that patients with abnormal hypopharyngeal reflux documented by pH monitoring were no more likely to respond to acid-suppressive therapy than patients with no documented reflux.[27] This raises the question as to whether these patients are suffering from excessive reflux or whether other diagnoses should be entertained. Overall, pH testing is valuable to suggest the presence or absence of reflux, but it does not suggest a causal link and, given its low sensitivity, it cannot be viewed as the gold standard in diagnosing LPR in patients referred for evaluation.

The role of pH and/or impedance monitoring in extraesophageal reflux (including LPR) is often to document normality rather than abnormal results. One important clinical question in the management of patients with extraesophageal reflux is if pH monitoring should be performed on or off of PPI therapy. The answer to this question is currently controversial, but the most recent study employing both impedance monitoring on therapy and wireless pH monitoring off of therapy suggests that a combined approach may be necessary.[28] Pritchett et al studied 39 patients with chronic throat symptoms with impedance/pH monitoring on twice-daily PPIs, and then the same patients were evaluated with wireless pH monitoring off of acid-suppressive therapy. The study showed that, on therapy, impedance testing was normal in 64% of patients; however, off of PPI therapy, it resulted in normal pH findings in only 28% of patients (Figure 4-4). Thus, in most patients with persistent throat symptoms on therapy, testing is more likely to exclude GER as the cause.[28] If impedance/pH testing is negative in these patients, a diagnosis other than reflux should be considered.

The current treatment recommendation for suspected extraesophageal reflux is aggressive acid-suppressive therapy empirically followed by testing (pH $\pm$ impedance and endoscopy).[29] Therapy response rates range from 60% to 98% in those with suspected LPR using a variety of antireflux treatments for varying durations.[1,7,18,30,31] The enthusiasm of treatment response in uncontrolled studies are, however, dampened by the overall undifferentiated response in controlled studies.[2,32-34] Accordingly, surgical studies suggest that there are poor surgical outcomes in patients unresponsive to medical treatment in this group of patients. So et al studied 150 patients after fundoplication and found that only 56% of patients had relief of extraesophageal symptoms, whereas 93% had improvement of heartburn.[35] More recently, Swoger et al evaluated the surgical response rate in a group of patients with LPR who were unresponsive to aggressive PPI therapy.[36] They studied 72 patients with symptoms consistent with LPR and treated them with 4 months of twice-daily PPI therapy. Twenty-five patients had less than 50% improvement despite maximal medical therapy. Ten of these patients underwent surgical fundoplication, while 15 remained on medical therapy alone. In the surgical group, one patient (10%) reported improvement in laryngeal symptoms at 1-year postoperation.[36]

The discussion that follows provides more detail into specific ENT diseases that have been associated with GER.

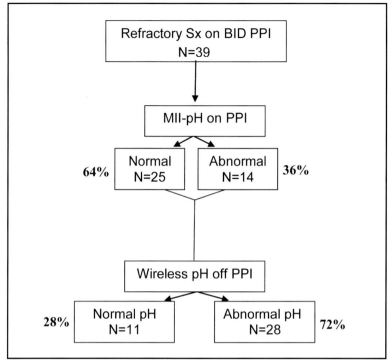

Figure 4-4. Flow diagram of likelihood of normal or abnormal impedance and wireless pH parameters in patients with refractory extraesophageal symptoms studied on therapy with impedance and off therapy with pH monitoring.

CHRONIC COUGH

Chronic cough is a very common complaint among outpatients. The most common causes are thought to be asthma, postnasal drip (PND), and reflux disease. Proposed mechanisms for cough by refluxate are stimulation of the afferent limb of the cough reflex by irritation of the upper respiratory tract without aspiration, irritation of the lower respiratory tract by either micro- or macroaspiration, and simulation of an esophageal-bronchial cough reflex.[37] Complicating matters is the evidence that cough might promote GER by causing transient lower esophageal sphincter relaxation or by increasing intrathoracic pressure in relation to intra-abdominal pressure.[38]

Esophageal pH monitoring has lower specificity for GER in patients with chronic cough.[37,39-41] In a combined pH and manometry evaluation performed by Paterson and Murat, only 1% of the total cough episodes per patient was associated with hypopharyngeal reflux events, on average.[42] However, given the discrete nature of cough episodes, recent studies have attempted to correlate timing of reflux events on pH or impedance monitoring with patients' report of cough spells. Sifrim and colleagues employed ambulatory pressure-pH-impedance monitoring with symptom association to assess the temporal association between cough and various constituents of reflux (acid, nonacid, liquid, or gas). They found that the majority of the cough events were not associated with reflux (highlighting causes other than GER), whereas 31% of the events were within the 2-minute time window of a reflux episode (either prior to the reflux or after). The nature of the refluxate in those with cough and reflux association were acidic in 65%, weakly acidic in 29%, and weakly alkaline 6% of the time.[43] The clinically important question, which is yet to be answered, is what role weakly acidic reflux plays in the persistence of cough in this group of patients. It is possible that impedance monitoring may be identifying a subgroup of people with chronic cough, possibly reflux related, who would not have been identified by pH monitoring alone; however, outcome studies are needed to be certain of this assertion.

It is intuitive that if acid reflux is playing a role in patients' cough, acid-suppressive therapy would be beneficial. A few studies suggest this possibility. In a retrospective study by Vaezi and Richter, 10 of 11 subjects with GER-related cough, who were subsequently treated with omeprazole as aggressive acid suppression, had complete resolution of coughing in less than 2 months.[39] In a double-blind, placebo-controlled study of pH recording performed by Kiljander et al, patients with both chronic cough and pathologic GER were randomized to placebo first and omeprazole second, or vice versa. Those who received placebo first with omeprazole second had a significant improvement in their cough score during the PPI treatment compared to baseline. In addition, although there was no statistically significant change initially in those who started on the omeprazole, at the end of the placebo period, the cough symptoms in the daytime improved significantly (p = 0.01). This suggests that the feedback loop between cough and GER might be suppressed with initial PPI treatment.[38] Waring et al, in their prospective study of those patients with both GER and chronic cough or hoarseness, found that if heartburn was eliminated with the addition of omeprazole, cough resolved in 9 of 16 patients (56%).[23] In another study to assess omeprazole response on chronic cough as a determinant of GER-induced cough, Ours and colleagues showed that treatment response could not be predicted by pH monitoring alone, as only 35% of those subjects with abnormal pH monitoring responded to omeprazole therapy.[40] Despite the above, seemingly positive studies suggest that PPI therapy might be beneficial in patients with chronic cough; other studies do not support a role for PPI therapy,[44] again highlighting the fact that in patients who do not respond to initial empiric PPI therapy, causes other than GER should be investigated.

CHRONIC LARYNGITIS

Chronic laryngitis is inflammation of the larynx that lasts more than a few weeks and is usually caused by an irritant, most commonly smoking. For patients who do not smoke, the next most commonly implicated cause may be reflux, often referred to as LPR. However, given that laryngeal response is similar to various irritants, laryngeal exam cannot specifically identify GER as the cause. Symptoms of LPR are nonspecific (see Table 4-1), and they include cough, throat clearing, sore throat, globus sensation, dysphonia, and dysphagia. These symptoms may occur due to injury of the structures of the larynx and pharynx, beginning with ciliary damage, which disrupts clearance function. Throat clearing is especially common among those with chronic laryngitis and can lead to worsening damage with repeated mechanical trauma.[45] The duration and severity of the symptoms of chronic laryngitis can vary widely among patients. The extent of laryngeal inflammation can also vary significantly. This variability again highlights the various causes for this condition. The most severe manifestation of chronic laryngitis may be ulceration of the epithelium with granulation.[45]

Initial studies in patients with LPR suggested increasing erythema and edema compared to the control population. For example, Hanson et al studied a group of patients with chronic posterior laryngitis and analyzed digital color images of the laryngeal exam in order to quantify the degree of erythema. The study found a significant difference in erythema among those with chronic laryngitis as compared to normal subjects, which reduced over time on antisecretory therapy (omeprazole).[46] However, this study was neither controlled nor blinded. More recent large-scale controlled studies suggest that

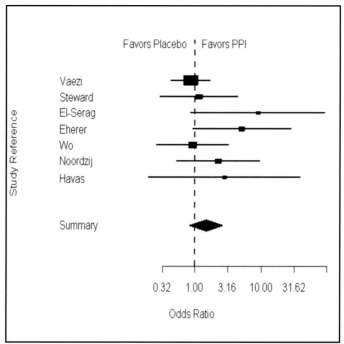

Figure 4-5. Forest plot depicting the odds ratio and 95% confidence intervals for studies assessing efficacy of PPI in reflux laryngitis.

laryngeal erythema and edema are nonspecific findings on laryngoscopy; can be found in healthy volunteers[9]; and are often associated with smoking, alcohol use, PND, and certain medication use. Thus, in a patient who is initially suspected of having GER-related laryngeal changes, lack of response to PPIs should prompt a search for nonreflux causes. This is further highlighted by the results of treatment studies in which, despite the initial favorable clinical response in small-scale uncontrolled studies,[30,45] the results of more recent placebo-controlled studies were disappointing. A meta-analysis of 8 pooled, randomized, controlled trials showed that treatment with PPIs did not lead to a significant improvement in symptoms for suspected GER-related chronic laryngitis (Figure 4-5). Only 1 of the 8 included studies showed a statistically significant effect prior to the meta-analysis, although 5 of the 8 showed a favorable but insignificant effect.[33] The largest multicenter study in 145 suspected LPR patients found no difference in symptoms or laryngeal sign resolution or improvement on esomeprazole 40 mg twice daily for 16 weeks compared to placebo (P = 0.799 and 0.466, respectively; see Figure 4-4).[47]

HOARSENESS

Underlying potential causes of chronic hoarseness include malignancy, vocal cord palsy, vocal cord lesions, laryngitis, functional disorders, and reflux disease. GER is suspected in up to 55% of patients with idiopathic hoarseness.[15] Multiple studies have assessed the treatment response with acid suppression, but a recent Cochrane review has demonstrated that few high-quality studies exist.[48] Prospective and retrospective studies show mixed results and there are no large-scale placebo-controlled studies assessing response to PPI therapy. In the study by Waring and colleagues, 8 out of 14 (57%) patients with improvement in heartburn had elimination of hoarseness.[23] However, given the multifactorial nature of the disease process, it is not unusual that patients often do not respond to PPI therapy. Impedance or pH monitoring in this group of patients is difficult to interpret since temporal association cannot be established between patients' symptoms and reflux events given the constant nature of hoarseness in general. Thus, it is reasonable to treat patients presenting with chronic hoarseness and benign laryngeal findings with a short course (2 months) of PPIs, especially if there is concomitant heartburn. If there is no clinical response, then a search for other potential causes would be prudent.

SINUSITIS

Chronic resistant sinusitis is defined by the presence of nasal symptoms, facial headache, and malaise for at least 6 weeks with objective evidence (by computed tomography or nasal endoscopy) of sinus disease. Chronic sinusitis becomes resistant when symptoms persist despite aggressive antibiotic therapy and sinus surgery.[49] The causes of chronic sinusitis are multifactorial and include infections, allergies, anatomic abnormalities of the sinuses/upper airway, and vasomotor reactivity that all lead to sinonasal edema.[49] Possible proposed mechanisms of GER contributing to sinusitis include inflammation-induced ostial obstruction, impaired mucociliary clearance secondary to acidic refluxate reaching the nasopharynx and posterior nasal passages, and reflux-induced autonomic nervous system hyperactivity leading to edema and obstruction or potentially due to *Helicobacter pylori* although little has been documented on this pathogen as a cause.[50,51]

A population-based study of a large group of veterans found that adults with complicated GER (evidence of esophagitis or esophageal stricture) were more likely than the controls to have sinusitis with an odds ratio of 1.60 (95% confidence interval [CI] 1.51 to 1.70).[52] Ulualp and Toohill compared 11 patients with chronic resistant sinusitis to healthy controls and found a significantly higher prevalence of pharyngeal acid reflux in the chronic resistant sinusitis group (64% versus 18%).[53] A small retrospective case series performed by DiBaise et al showed an association between chronic sinusitis and GER, but the causal link could not be assessed.[54] In patients postsinus surgery, preoperative presence of GER, defined as the presence of heartburn or regurgitation, was a significant predictor of poor symptom outcome following sinus surgery.[55] In a different study, DiBaise et al showed a high prevalence of GER in patients with chronic resistant sinusitis. The study demonstrated a modest improvement in facial headache and sinus pressure using twice-daily omeprazole for 3 months.[49] In a prospective study, DelGaudio showed that not only does the chronic resistant sinusitis group have more reflux symptoms, but that the amount of nasopharyngeal reflux events were also more common in the chronic resistant sinusitis group as compared to controls (39% compared to 10% and 5%, respectively, with a P = 0.01).[51] In direct contrast, a similar study by Jecker and colleagues of patients with chronic polypoid rhinosinusitis, who underwent both esophageal and hypopharyngeal pH monitoring, demonstrated that the number of hypopharyngeal reflux events was not significantly different than in controls, suggesting that chronic resistant sinusitis may not be associated with direct acid injury.[56] Thus, the association between GER and chronic resistant sinusitis remains controversial.

POSTNASAL DRIP

PND occurs with excessive mucus production, or impaired mucociliary clearance, resulting in the sensation of drainage, chronic throat clearing, and irritation. In many patients, PND coexists with sinonasal allergy and/or chronic sinusitis. PND has been associated with GER; however, similar to other extraesophageal symptoms, the causal link has been difficult to establish. There is a scarcity of clinical studies in regard to GER and PND; however, the most recent studies show promise on the clinical response of patients to acid-suppressive therapy. In a study by Pawar et al, patients with PND (but no evidence of sinonasal disease) were randomized to PPI therapy versus no therapy. PPI therapy improved the frequency of PND, but there was no significant difference in improvement in the reflux symptom index.[57] The most recent placebo-controlled study by Vaezi et al suggested significant benefit to PPI therapy in this group of difficult-to-treat patients. In this study, 75 patients with chronic isolated PND (but no significant allergies) were randomized to 4 months of lansoprazole 30 mg twice daily or placebo for 4 months. Symptom improvement was assessed by a GER quality of life instrument and PND was assessed by RSOM31 and SNOT 20 validated questionnaires. At 2 and 4 months post-therapy, significantly more improvement was noted in the group on PPI therapy than controls, suggesting a possible link between GER and PND.[58]

OTITIS MEDIA

Otitis media (OM) has also been implicated as a possible disease process related to GER. The pathogenesis relates to eustachian tube dysfunction associated with the entry of fluids from the nasopharynx into the middle ear by reflux. Such fluid would then cause inflammation leading to increased mucus production, mucociliary impairment, and ultimately an impaired ability to equalize middle ear pressure.[59] In a study by Heavner et al, eustachian tubes of rats exposed to pepsin and HCl had elevated passive opening pressures as well as decreased ability to clear both positive and negative pressure. Repeat exposures over time showed worsening ability of the eustachian tube to clear positive or negative pressure.[60] In human subjects, the association with subjective GER symptoms and detection of pepsin has been mixed. A questionnaire study by Lieu et al did not find a correlation between reflux symptoms and elevated pepsin or pepsinogen I aspirated from middle ear fluid.[61] In another study, pepsinogen levels in the effusions were significantly higher in patients with than without GER. In addition, the patients treated for reflux with PPIs had decreased pepsinogen levels in their middle ear effusions.[62] In one prospective pediatric study, GER was present in 64% of the study group (those with OM with effusions) and pharyngeal reflux was documented in 48% of children with OM versus 25% and 8.3% in the control groups, respectively (P < 0.05).[63] The majority of studies of GER and OM is in the pediatric population and most are case series and uncontrolled, hence the true causal relationship awaits future controlled studies.

LARYNGEAL CANCER

Laryngeal cancer is one of the most common head and neck cancers in the United States with an annual incidence estimated to be approximately 12,000 new cases per year. The 5-year relative survival rate is approximately 64%.[64] The role of GER in laryngeal cancer is currently controversial. GER is implicated in some due to its high prevalence in those with laryngeal carcinoma. However, this relationship is confounded by the association between GER and smoking and alcohol use, the 2 most common etiologies for laryngeal cancer. Most studies in this area suffer from lack of an acceptable control group and they do not control for the interaction between GER and alcohol and tobacco use.[65]

In a case-control study of veterans, GER was associated with laryngeal cancer with an adjusted odds ratio of 2.40 among hospitalized patients (95% CI 2.15 to 2.69, p < 0.0001) and 2.31 (95% CI 2.10 to 2.53, p < 0.0001) for outpatients.[66] In contrast, Geterud and colleagues compared pH monitoring data in subjects with recently diagnosed laryngeal carcinoma

Table 4-3					Case Control Studies on Laryngeal Cancer and GERD*			
STUDY AUTHOR	# OF CASES	# OF CONTROLS	GERD IN CASES	GERD IN CONTROLS	SMOKING (CASES/ CONTROLS)	ALCOHOL (CASES/ CONTROLS)	ODDS RATIO (95% CI)	% RANDOM EFFECTS WEIGHTS
El-Serag[66]	17520	70080	3634 (21%)	5855 (8%)	(+/+)	(+/+)	2.87 (2.74 to 3.00)	32.98
Koufman[1]	31	151	22 (71%)	91 (60%)	(+/+)	(–/–)	1.61 (0.69 to 3.74)	18.35
Chen[65]	63	735	34 (54%)	365 (50%)	(+/–)	(–/–)	1.19 (0.71 to 1.99)	25.40
Mercante[69]	92	636	20 (25%)	32 (5%)	NS/NS	(–/–)	5.24 (2.85 to 9.65)	23.26

*With respect to patient distribution, GERD prevalence, evaluation of confounding risk factors, calculated odds, ratio, and effective weight of each study on overall model.

Pooled odds ratio by random effects model: 2.37 (1.38 to 4.08).

(+) Indicates risk factor was evaluated and (–) indicates that the risk factor was not evaluated in the study. NS indicates nonsmokers.

The weights determine the influence of each study on the combined results.

and controls finding no difference in the mean acid exposure time or number of reflux events.[67] Similarly, a meta-analysis by Qadeer et al, analyzing 4 case-control studies, found that GER prevalence was nearly 2 times higher in the patients with laryngeal carcinoma than controls (Table 4-3). This increased prevalence was especially evident in evaluated studies with nonsmoking and nonalcohol-consuming subjects with laryngeal cancer, indicating a potential relationship independent of tobacco or alcohol use.[68-70] In a recent case-control study by Vaezi and colleagues in which patients were matched by age, gender, and ethnicity, smoking and GER were significant risk factors for the development of laryngeal cancer. GER was significantly associated in both the univariable and multivariable models with odds ratios of 1.79 (95% CI 1.03 to 3.11) and 2.11 (95% CI 1.16 to 3.85), respectively. In addition, symptomatic GER was more frequent in patients with laryngeal cancer compared to controls. Although this study does not prove causality, it does point toward a possible link between the 2 conditions.[71]

POSTVIRAL VOCAL CORD DYSFUNCTION

Vocal cord dysfunction (VCD) or paradoxical vocal fold dysfunction (PVFD) is a disorder of the larynx in which the vocal cords inappropriately adduct during inspiration, causing partial and possibly severe airflow obstruction. It is often misdiagnosed as asthma. Possible proposed mechanisms of the disorder include caustic irritants (GER, PND, or inhaled particles) leading to a maladaptive response for airway protection, cortical injury involving upper or lower motor neurons, or increased autonomic tone leading to inappropriate closure. Another theory is that the response is a type of conversion response from an underlying psychiatric condition.[72] Initial case reports suggested an association with upper respiratory infections and VCD; however, this association has not been confirmed.[72-74]

A case-control study by Perkner et al described 11 cases of irritant-associated VCD and compared them to nonexposed VCD subjects. In this study, there was a high rate of GER (described as symptoms of indigestion, retrosternal burning, waterbrash, or objective evidence of reflux by pH) in both groups at 70% and 59% in the irritant and nonirritant VCD groups, respectively.[75] In another case series of 5 subjects with refractory cough and PVFD, acid-suppressive therapy did not result in symptom improvement while respiratory retraining was successful in improving patients' cough.[74] Thus, given the paucity of data and lack of large-scale controlled studies, the association between VCD and GER remains uncertain, and PPI use can only be advocated in those with concomitant heartburn.

SUBGLOTTIC STENOSIS

Laryngeal stenosis most often occurs in patients with trauma from intubation. Concomitant GER may result in poor healing and resistant stenosis. Most commonly laryngeal stenosis occurs in the posterior commissure and subglottic areas.[76] GER is implicated in idiopathic subglottic stenosis where patients do not have a history of tracheal intubation. Walner et al evaluated esophageal pH data in children with subglottic stenosis reporting a significant number of reflux events; however, the study was retrospective, uncontrolled, and observational in nature.[77] In a study of a large veterans' database, El-Serag and Sonnenberg found that subjects with complicated GER were more likely to have laryngeal stenosis with an odds ratio of 2.02 (95% CI 1.12 to 3.65).[52] In Koufman's study, 10 of 15 patients with stenosis were found to have abnormal pharyngeal pH studies. In addition, the highest rate of abnormality with both esophageal and pharyngeal reflux was in those not treated with antireflux therapy prior to the study.[1] However, most studies suggesting a link between GER and subglottic stenosis are uncontrolled and observational in nature. While awaiting more definitive studies, empiric therapy with PPIs may be reasonable in those with baseline symptoms of heartburn and/or regurgitation.

CONCLUSION

The association between laryngeal disease and GER is clearly documented not only based on observational but also controlled trials. The strength of evidence is varied among different laryngeal symptoms (Table 4-4). Controversy exists regarding the appropriate diagnostic methodology and therefore the true frequency of GER as the causal etiology in many who do not respond to aggressive acid suppression. Laryngeal examination lacks specificity and pH monitoring lacks sensitivity in establishing a true link. Thus, until more definitive tests are available, the current recommendations in this group of patients would be a trial of twice-daily PPI therapy for approximately 2 months (Figure 4-6). If the patient fails to respond, pH with or without impedance monitoring is the appropriate initial diagnostic strategy to rule out continued acidic or nonacidic reflux. Endoscopy in general has low clinical yield and is recommended only in those presenting with warning symptoms such as dysphagia, chest pain, odynophagia, weight loss, or anemia. In patients who do not respond to aggressive acid suppression and have normal pH or impedance, a search should

Table 4-4	Quality of Evidence for Association of GERD
Chronic cough	Fair
Chronic laryngitis	Fair
Hoarseness	Poor
Sinusitis	Fair
Postnasal drip	Good
Otitis media	Poor
Laryngeal cancer	Fair
Postviral vocal cord dysfunction	Poor
Subglottic stenosis	Poor

Good: Evidence includes consistent results from well-designed, well-conducted studies in representative populations that directly assess effects on health outcomes.

Fair: Evidence is sufficient to determine effects on health outcomes, but the strength of the evidence is limited by the number, quality, or consistency of the individual studies, generalizability to routine practice, or indirect nature of the evidence on health outcomes.

Poor: Evidence is insufficient to assess the effects on health outcomes because of limited number or power of studies, important flaws in their design or conduct, gaps in the chain of evidence, or lack of information on important health outcomes.

Figure 4-6. Treatment algorithm for suspected GER-related extraesophageal symptoms.

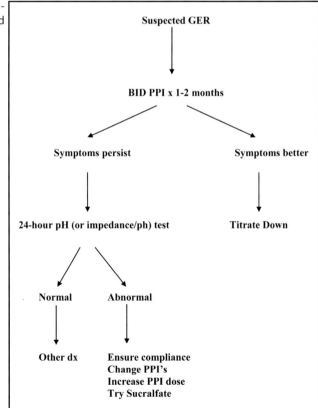

be initiated for potential other causes for patients' continued symptoms. Surgical therapy may be a consideration only in those responsive to therapy but requiring high doses of acid suppression, continued regurgitation, cost of the medication, or with potential side effects to medical therapy.

REFERENCES

1. Koufman JA. The otolaryngologic manifestations of gastroesophageal reflux disease (GERD): a clinical investigation of 225 patients using ambulatory 24-hour pH monitoring and an experimental investigation of the role of acid and pepsin in the development of laryngeal injury. *Laryngoscope.* 1991;101(4 pt 2 suppl 53):1-78.
2. Vaezi MF, Hicks DM, Abelson TI, Richter JE. Laryngeal signs and symptoms and gastroesophageal reflux disease (GERD): a critical assessment of cause and effect association. *Clin Gastroenterol Hepatol.* 2003;1(5):333-344.
3. DeVault KR. Extraesophageal symptoms of GERD. *Cleve Clin J Med.* 2003;70(suppl 5):S20-S32.
4. Delahunty JE, Cherry J. Experimentally produced vocal cord granulomas. *Laryngoscope.* 1968;78(11):1941-1947.
5. Little FB, Koufman JA, Kohut RI, Marshall RB. Effect of gastric acid on the pathogenesis of subglottic stenosis. *Ann Otol Rhinol Laryngol.* 1985;94(5 pt 1):516-519. Abstract.
6. Adhami T, Goldblum JR, Richter JE, Vaezi MF. The role of gastric and duodenal agents in laryngeal injury: an experimental canine model. *Am J Gastroenterol.* 2004;99(11):2098-2106.
7. Vaezi MF. Sensitivity and specificity of reflux-attributed laryngeal lesions: experimental and clinical evidence. *Am J Med.* 2003;115(suppl 3A):97S-104S.
8. Heidelbaugh JJ, Gill AS, Van Harrison R, Nostrant TT. Atypical presentations of gastroesophageal reflux disease. *Am Fam Physician.* 2008;78(4):483-488.
9. Hicks DM, Ours TM, Abelson TI, Vaezi MF, Richter JE. The prevalence of hypopharynx findings associated with gastroesophageal reflux in normal volunteers. *J Voice.* 2002;16(4):564-579.
10. Vavricka SR, Storck CA, Wildi SM, et al. Limited diagnostic value of laryngopharyngeal lesions in patients with gastroesophageal reflux during routine upper gastrointestinal endoscopy. *Am J Gastroenterol.* 2007;102(4):716-722.
11. Qadeer MA, Swoger J, Milstein C, et al. Correlation between symptoms and laryngeal signs in laryngopharyngeal reflux. *Laryngoscope.* 2005;115(11):1947-1952.
12. Ahmed TF, Khandwala F, Abelson TI, et al. Chronic laryngitis associated with gastroesophageal reflux: prospective assessment of differences in practice patterns between gastroenterologists and ENT physicians. *Am J Gastroenterol.* 2006;101(3):470-478.
13. Sermon F, Vanden Brande S, Roosens B, Mana F, Deron P, Urbain D. Is ambulatory 24-h dual-probe pH monitoring useful in suspected ENT manifestations of GERD? *Dig Liver Dis.* 2004;36(2):105-110.
14. Baldi F, Cappiello R, Cavoli C, Ghersi S, Torresan F, Roda E. Proton pump inhibitor treatment of patients with gastroesophageal reflux-related chronic cough: a comparison between two different daily doses of lansoprazole. *World J Gastroenterol.* 2006;12(1):82-88.
15. McNally PR, Maydonovitch CL, Prosek RA, Collette RP, Wong RK. Evaluation of gastroesophageal reflux as a cause of idiopathic hoarseness. *Dig Dis Sci.* 1989;34(12):1900-1904.
16. Wiener GJ, Koufman JA, Wu WC, Cooper JB, Richter JE, Castell DO. Chronic hoarseness secondary to gastroesophageal reflux disease: documentation with 24-h ambulatory pH monitoring. *Am J Gastroenterol.* 1989;84(12):1503-1508.
17. Vaezi MF, Schroeder PL, Richter JE. Reproducibility of proximal probe pH parameters in 24-hour ambulatory esophageal pH monitoring. *Am J Gastroenterol.* 1997;92(5):825-829.
18. Park W, Hicks DM, Khandwala F, et al. Laryngopharyngeal reflux: prospective cohort study evaluating optimal dose of proton-pump inhibitor therapy and pretherapy predictors of response. *Laryngoscope.* 2005;115(7):1230-1238.
19. Bardan E. Pharyngoesophageal pH monitoring. *Am J Med.* 2003;115(suppl 3A):78S-80S.
20. Jamieson JR, Stein HJ, DeMeester TR, et al. Ambulatory 24-h esophageal pH monitoring: normal values, optimal thresholds, specificity, sensitivity, and reproducibility. *Am J Gastroenterol.* 1992;87(9):1102-1111.
21. Reichel O, Issing WJ. Impact of different pH thresholds for 24-hour dual probe pH monitoring in patients with suspected laryngopharyngeal reflux. *J Laryngol Otol.* 2008;122(5):485-489.
22. Shaker R, Milbrath M, Ren J, et al. Esophagopharyngeal distribution of refluxed gastric acid in patients with reflux laryngitis. *Gastroenterology.* 1995;109(5):1575-1582.

23. Waring JP, Lacayo L, Hunter J, Katz E, Suwak B. Chronic cough and hoarseness in patients with severe gastroesophageal reflux disease. Diagnosis and response to therapy. *Dig Dis Sci.* 1995;40(5):1093-1097.

24. Jacob P, Kahrilas PJ, Herzon G. Proximal esophageal pH-metry in patients with 'reflux laryngitis.' *Gastroenterology.* 1991;100(2):305-310.

25. Eubanks TR, Omelanczuk PE, Maronian N, Hillel A, Pope CE 2nd, Pellegrini CA. Pharyngeal pH monitoring in 222 patients with suspected laryngeal reflux. *J Gastrointest Surg.* 2001;5(2):183-190; discussion 190-191.

26. Vaezi MF. Gastroesophageal reflux disease and the larynx. *J Clin Gastroenterol.* 2003;36(3):198-203.

27. Ulualp SO, Toohill RJ, Shaker R. Outcomes of acid suppressive therapy in patients with posterior laryngitis. *Otolaryngol Head Neck Surg.* 2001;124(1):16-22.

28. Pritchett JM, Aslam M, Slaughter JC, Ness RM, Garrett CG, Vaezi MF. Efficacy of esophageal impedance/pH monitoring in patients with refractory gastroesophageal reflux disease, on and off therapy. *Clin Gastroenterol Hepatol.* 2009;7(7):743-748.

29. Kahrilas PJ, Shaheen NJ, Vaezi MF. American Gastroenterological Association Institute technical review on the management of gastroesophageal reflux disease. *Gastroenterology.* 2008;135(4):1392-1413.

30. Hanson DG, Kamel PL, Kahrilas PJ. Outcomes of antireflux therapy for the treatment of chronic laryngitis. *Ann Otol Rhinol Laryngol.* 1995;104(7):550-555. Abstract.

31. Kamel PL, Hanson D, Kahrilas PJ. Omeprazole for the treatment of posterior laryngitis. *Am J Med.* 1994;96(4):321-326. Abstract.

32. Karkos PD, Wilson JA. Empiric treatment of laryngopharyngeal reflux with proton pump inhibitors: a systematic review. *Laryngoscope.* 2006;116(1):144-148.

33. Qadeer MA, Phillips CO, Lopez AR, et al. Proton pump inhibitor therapy for suspected GERD-related chronic laryngitis: a meta-analysis of randomized controlled trials. *Am J Gastroenterol.* 2006;101(11):2646-2654.

34. Mastronarde JG, Anthonisen NR, Castro M, et al. Efficacy of esomeprazole for treatment of poorly controlled asthma. *N Engl J Med.* 2009;360(15):1487-1499.

35. So JB, Zeitels SM, Rattner DW. Outcomes of atypical symptoms attributed to gastroesophageal reflux treated by laparoscopic fundoplication. *Surgery.* 1998;124(1):28-32.

36. Swoger J, Ponsky J, Hicks DM, et al. Surgical fundoplication in laryngopharyngeal reflux unresponsive to aggressive acid suppression: a controlled study. *Clin Gastroenterol Hepatol.* 2006;4(4):433-441.

37. Irwin RS. Chronic cough due to gastroesophageal reflux disease: ACCP evidence-based clinical practice guidelines. *Chest.* 2006;129(1 suppl):80S-94S.

38. Kiljander TO, Salomaa ER, Hietanen EK, Terho EO. Chronic cough and gastro-oesophageal reflux: a double-blind placebo-controlled study with omeprazole. *Eur Respir J.* 2000;16(4):633-638.

39. Vaezi MF, Richter JE. Twenty-four-hour ambulatory esophageal pH monitoring in the diagnosis of acid reflux-related chronic cough. *South Med J.* 1997;90(3):305-311.

40. Ours TM, Kavuru MS, Schilz RJ, Richter JE. A prospective evaluation of esophageal testing and a double-blind, randomized study of omeprazole in a diagnostic and therapeutic algorithm for chronic cough. *Am J Gastroenterol.* 1999;94(11):3131-3138.

41. Frye JW, Vaezi MF. Extraesophageal GERD. *Gastroenterol Clin North Am.* 2008;37(4):845-858, ix.

42. Paterson WG, Murat BW. Combined ambulatory esophageal manometry and dual-probe pH-metry in evaluation of patients with chronic unexplained cough. *Dig Dis Sci.* 1994;39(5):1117-1125.

43. Sifrim D, Dupont L, Blondeau K, Zhang X, Tack J, Janssens J. Weakly acidic reflux in patients with chronic unexplained cough during 24 hour pressure, pH, and impedance monitoring. *Gut.* 2005;54(4):449-454.

44. Chang AB, Lasserson TJ, Kiljander TO, Connor FL, Gaffney JT, Garske LA. Systematic review and meta-analysis of randomised controlled trials of gastro-oesophageal reflux interventions for chronic cough associated with gastro-oesophageal reflux. *Br Med J.* 2006;332(7532):11-17.

45. Hanson DG, Jiang JJ. Diagnosis and management of chronic laryngitis associated with reflux. *Am J Med.* 2000;108(suppl 4a):112S-119S.

46. Hanson DG, Jiang J, Chi W. Quantitative color analysis of laryngeal erythema in chronic posterior laryngitis. *J Voice.* 1998;12(1):78-83.

47. Vaezi MF, Richter JE, Stasney CR, et al. Treatment of chronic posterior laryngitis with esomeprazole. *Laryngoscope.* 2006;116(2):254-260.

48. Hopkins C, Yousaf U, Pedersen M. Acid reflux treatment for hoarseness. *Cochrane Database Syst Rev.* 2006;(1):CD005054.

49. DiBaise JK, Olusola BF, Huerter JV, Quigley EM. Role of GERD in chronic resistant sinusitis: a prospective, open label, pilot trial. *Am J Gastroenterol.* 2002;97(4):843-850.

50. Ulualp SO, Toohill RJ, Hoffmann R, Shaker R. Possible relationship of gastroesophagopharyngeal acid reflux with pathogenesis of chronic sinusitis. *Am J Rhinol.* 1999;13(3):197-202.

51. DelGaudio JM. Direct nasopharyngeal reflux of gastric acid is a contributing factor in refractory chronic rhinosinusitis. *Laryngoscope.* 2005;115(6):946-957.

52. El-Serag HB, Sonnenberg A. Comorbid occurrence of laryngeal or pulmonary disease with esophagitis in United States military veterans. *Gastroenterology.* 1997;113(3):755-760.

53. Ulualp SO, Toohill RJ. Laryngopharyngeal reflux: state of the art diagnosis and treatment. *Otolaryngol Clin North Am.* 2000;33(4):785-802.

54. DiBaise JK, Huerter JV, Quigley EM. Sinusitis and gastroesophageal reflux disease. *Ann Intern Med.* 1998;129(12):1078.

55. Chambers DW, Davis WE, Cook PR, Nishioka GJ, Rudman DT. Long-term outcome analysis of functional endoscopic sinus surgery: correlation of symptoms with endoscopic examination findings and potential prognostic variables. *Laryngoscope.* 1997;107(4):504-510.

56. Jecker P, Orloff LA, Wohlfeil M, Mann WJ. Gastroesophageal reflux disease (GERD), extraesophageal reflux (EER) and recurrent chronic rhinosinusitis. *Eur Arch Otorhinolaryngol.* 2006;263(7):664-667.

57. Pawar S, Lim HJ, Gill M, et al. Treatment of postnasal drip with proton pump inhibitors: a prospective, randomized, placebo-controlled study. *Am J Rhinol.* 2007;21(6):695-701.

58. Vaezi M HD, Slaughter JC, Tanner SB, et al. A randomized double-blind placebo-controlled study of acid suppression for isolated chronic postnasal drip. *Gastroenterology.* 2009;136(5):A-685.

59. Schreiber S, Garten D, Sudhoff H. Pathophysiological mechanisms of extraesophageal reflux in otolaryngeal disorders. *Eur Arch Otorhinolaryngol.* 2009;266(1):17-24.

60. Heavner SB, Hardy SM, White DR, McQueen CT, Prazma J, Pillsbury HC 3rd. Function of the eustachian tube after weekly exposure to pepsin/hydrochloric acid. *Otolaryngol Head Neck Surg.* 2001;125(3):123-129.

61. Lieu JE, Muthappan PG, Uppaluri R. Association of reflux with otitis media in children. *Otolaryngol Head Neck Surg.* 2005;133(3):357-361.

62. Sone M, Yamamuro Y, Hayashi H, Niwa Y, Nakashima T. Otitis media in adults as a symptom of gastroesophageal reflux. *Otolaryngol Head Neck Surg.* 2007;136(1):19-22.

63. Keles B, Ozturk K, Gunel E, Arbag H, Ozer B. Pharyngeal reflux in children with chronic otitis media with effusion. *Acta Otolaryngol.* 2004;124(10):1178-1181.

64. Jemal A, Siegel R, Ward E, Hao Y, Xu J, Thun MJ. Cancer statistics, 2009. *CA Cancer J Clin.* 2009;59(4):225-249.

65. Qadeer MA, Colabianchi N, Strome M, Vaezi MF. Gastroesophageal reflux and laryngeal cancer: causation or association? A critical review. *Am J Otolaryngol.* 2006;27(2):119-128.

66. El-Serag HB, Hepworth EJ, Lee P, Sonnenberg A. Gastroesophageal reflux disease is a risk factor for laryngeal and pharyngeal cancer. *Am J Gastroenterol.* 2001;96(7):2013-2018.

67. Geterud A, Bove M, Ruth M. Hypopharyngeal acid exposure: an independent risk factor for laryngeal cancer? *Laryngoscope.* 2003;113(12):2201-2205.

68. Qadeer MA, Colabianchi N, Vaezi MF. Is GERD a risk factor for laryngeal cancer? *Laryngoscope.* 2005;115(3):486-491.

69. Mercante G, Bacciu A, Ferri T, Bacciu S. Gastroesophageal reflux as a possible co-promoting factor in the development of the squamous-cell carcinoma of the oral cavity, of the larynx and of the pharynx. *Acta Otorhinolaryngol Belg.* 2003;57(2):113-117. Abstract.

70. Morrison MD. Is chronic gastroesophageal reflux a causative factor in glottic carcinoma? *Otolaryngol Head Neck Surg.* 1988;99(4):370-373. Abstract.

71. Vaezi MF, Qadeer MA, Lopez R, Colabianchi N. Laryngeal cancer and gastroesophageal reflux disease: a case-control study. *Am J Med.* 2006;119(9):768-776.

72. Mikita JA, Mikita CP. Vocal cord dysfunction. *Allergy Asthma Proc.* 2006;27(4):411-414.

73. Kellman RM, Leopold DA. Paradoxical vocal cord motion: an important cause of stridor. *Laryngoscope.* 1982;92(1):58-60.

74. Murry T, Tabaee A, Aviv JE. Respiratory retraining of refractory cough and laryngopharyngeal reflux in patients with paradoxical vocal fold movement disorder. *Laryngoscope.* 2004;114(8):1341-1345.

75. Perkner JJ, Fennelly KP, Balkissoon R, et al. Irritant-associated vocal cord dysfunction. *J Occup Environ Med.* 1998;40(2):136-143.

76. Toohill RJ, Kuhn JC. Role of refluxed acid in pathogenesis of laryngeal disorders. *Am J Med.* 1997;103(suppl 5A):100S-106S.

77. Walner DL, Stern Y, Gerber ME, Rudolph C, Baldwin CY, Cotton RT. Gastroesophageal reflux in patients with subglottic stenosis. *Arch Otolaryngol Head Neck Surg.* 1998;124(5):551-555.

Editorial: Point Counterpoint

Anthony J. DiMarino Jr, MD and Sidney Cohen, MD

LPR, also known as reflux laryngitis or GER-related laryngitis, has historically been a topic of controversy between otolaryngologists and gastroenterologists. The diagnosis of LPR requires multiple office visits and invasive diagnostic tests. Acid-suppressive medications are the first-line therapeutic agents in the treatment of LPR and account for a significant proportion of health care expenditures in United States. In this chapter, we reviewed the otolaryngologist (Spiegel) and the gastroenterologist perspective (Cassani and Vaezi) on this disorder, which has a significant impact on the utilization of health care in this country. Both perspectives agree on the evidence that is currently available for evaluating the association between different clinical manifestations of LPR and GER.

In clinical practice, it is often hard to differentiate GER from other causative factors (eg, smoking, allergens, or pollutants). Spiegel mentions that, after careful history taking, otolaryngologists often consider LPR a primary cause of common symptoms of laryngeal and throat irritation and a secondary cause of more distant chronic inflammation in the nose, paranasal sinuses, and the middle ear. Cassani and Vaezi have carefully evaluated the current evidence behind this common practice (see Table 4-4) and conclude that the quality of evidence regarding the association of GER with chronic cough, laryngitis, and sinusitis is fair. There is good evidence regarding the association of GER with PND. It is important to note that association does not indicate causation, and clinicians should carefully set therapeutic goals and endpoints before treating patients.

Laryngeal cancer is a common head and neck malignancy encountered in otolaryngology practice. Studies have shown a significant association between symptomatic and asymptomatic GER and the presence of laryngeal cancer. Even though it is difficult to establish a causal relationship, we agree with Speigel's recommendation regarding the use of acid suppression in patients with premalignant laryngeal disorders and those undergoing treatment for laryngeal cancer.

Otolaryngologists are the primary contact for patients presenting with laryngeal symptoms and depend on laryngoscopy to make the initial diagnosis. Due to the poor specificity of largyngoscopic findings, patients often undergo further testing in the form of pH/impendance testing and/or esophagoscopy. Unfortunately, as mentioned by Vaezi, the tools available to gastroenterologists have poor sensitivity at diagnosing GER associated with LPR and often fail to establish a causal relationship.

The currently established clinical practice recommendations are to treat patients suspected of having LPR with 2 to 4 months of twice-daily PPI therapy (see Figure 4-6). As indicated by Spiegel, it is important to define the symptoms treated and monitor for improvement and compliance. In patients who fail to improve with this therapy and have normal esophageal pH on therapy, therapy should be discontinued and other diagnoses should be considered.

chapter 5

Sleep Disturbance and Esophageal Reflux

Christine Herdman, MD; Dina Halegoua-DeMarzio, MD;
Sidney Cohen, MD; and Anthony J. DiMarino Jr, MD

Gastroesophageal reflux disease (GERD) is a chronic disorder of the esophagus with a spectrum of symptoms including heartburn and regurgitation. It has been estimated that 7% of individuals in the general population experience symptoms of this disease daily, and 14% have GERD symptoms at least once a week.[1] Nocturnal GERD occurs when gastric contents reflux into the esophagus while an individual is in a recumbent state. In 2000, the Gallup Organization, on behalf of the American Gastroenterological Association, conducted a nationwide telephone survey of 1000 adults experiencing heartburn at least once a week to help determine the impact of nighttime heartburn on sleep. Of these respondents, 79% reported heartburn at night and 75% reported that the symptoms affected their sleep.[2]

Beyond being a common and bothersome disease, nocturnal acid reflux has been associated with severe reflux-induced injuries including erosion, esophagitis, strictures, Barrett's esophagus, and perhaps adenocarcinoma due to direct and prolonged esophageal acid exposure.[3-6] The relationship between sleep and GERD is further complicated by interesting data in which patients with self-described insomnia and no known history of GERD had improved sleep efficiency when administered a proton pump inhibitor (PPI).[7] The necessity of sleep makes sleep disturbance a very important extraesophageal manifestation of GERD. This chapter will further evaluate the complex relationship between sleep and GERD.

PREVALENCE OF SLEEP DISTURBANCE AMONG PATIENTS WITH GERD

Although a large body of information exists about the prevalence of GERD in general, data specifically addressing the frequency and severity of nocturnal GERD are limited. It is now recognized that the majority of GERD patients experience nocturnal symptoms.

DiMarino AJ Jr, Cohen S, eds.
Extraesophageal Manifestations of GERD (pp 75-82).
© 2013 Taylor & Francis Group.

As stated previously, in a study utilizing the Gallup survey, 79% of respondents reported heartburn at night and 75% had symptoms that affected their sleep.[2] In addition to affecting sleep, 40% of respondents also noted that nocturnal heartburn adversely affected their daily activity. Thirty-four percent of the patients reported sleeping upright or in a chair due to nocturnal heartburn symptoms and 39% took naps whenever possible. In a study based on data from the 2006 US National Health and Wellness Survey, Mody et al identified 11,685 respondents with GERD. In this study, 88.9% of respondents experienced nighttime symptoms, 68.3% reported sleep difficulties, 49.1% had difficulty initiating asleep, and 58.3% had difficulty maintaining sleep.[8]

Respondents with nighttime GERD symptoms differed from those without nighttime symptoms in that they tend to be younger, more likely to smoke, and more likely to experience a psychiatric comorbidity. Other predictors of nocturnal reflux as determined by the Sleep Heart Health Study[9] include the following:

- Increased body mass index
- Carbonated soft drink consumption
- Snoring and daytime sleepiness
- Insomnia
- Hypertension
- Asthma
- Use of benzodiazepines

In addition, those respondents with sleep difficulties sought more significant health care resources including emergency room visits, hospitalization, and office visits. With regard to work productivity, respondents with GERD-related sleep difficulties reported greater absenteeism and overall work impairment.[8,9] Based on these and other epidemiologic studies,[8-10] it is obvious that GERD-related sleep disturbance has a significant impact on quality of life, work productivity, and the utilization of health care resources. Given the financial impact and effect on quality of life, it is important to investigate and clarify the pathophysiology of nocturnal reflux and its relationship to sleep disturbance.

PATHOPHYSIOLOGY OF THE LINK BETWEEN SLEEP DISTURBANCE AND GERD

The mechanism between nighttime GERD and sleep disturbance is not clearly unidirectional or bidirectional. The state of sleep is associated with a decrease in swallowing, subsequent reduced amounts of salivary bicarbonate, and reduced esophageal peristalsis and gravity. All of these factors can increase the severity and amount of refluxate. Sleep deprivation itself has been associated with increased perception and reported GERD symptoms.[11] In healthy individuals, nocturnal acid reflux results in sleep arousal or awakening, which leads to a swallow reflex. When the esophagus comes into contact with acid, there is an increase in salivary flow. The swallowing mechanism initiates peristalsis, which results in the neutralization of esophageal contents with bicarbonate-rich saliva. Swallowing frequency is greatly decreased during sleep; swallows only occur during brief arousals. Salivary secretion ceases during sleep, and sleep facilitates proximal acid migration into the esophagus.[12] Arousals and awakenings from sleep facilitate esophageal acid clearance but can lead to sleep disturbance (Figure 5-1).

In a study by Orr et al, it was demonstrated that the infusion of acid into the normal subject provoked an arousal from sleep greater than the infusion of water.[13] The higher

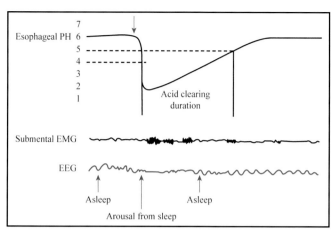

Figure 5-1. Infusion of acid into the normal subject provokes an arousal from sleep. (Adapted from Orr WC, Robinson MG, Johnson LF. The effect of esophageal acid volume on arousals from sleep and acid clearance. *Chest.* 1991;99:351-354.)

the level of wakefulness, as detected by polysomnography, the more rapid the acid clearance. Peristaltic parameters were not different during acid versus water infusions or by sleep versus waking stages. In a follow-up evaluation, Orr and colleagues showed that the latency to arousal was much shorter with a greater volume of acid infused during sleep. It was proposed that the larger volume provided a "warning signal" to the central nervous system, which leads to arousal. While awake, the volume did not affect latency to first swallow.[14,15]

The average acid contact time during sleep is between approximately 1.2% and 2%. In comparison, the average acid contact time during daytime and upright positions is approximately 6% to 8% in healthy volunteers without mucosal damage or complaints of heartburn. Esophageal pH monitoring is the current gold standard for diagnosing GERD. It provides direct physiologic measurement of acid in the esophagus and is the most objective method to document and assess the severity of the disease. The severity of GERD is determined by a DeMeester score, which takes into account 6 different parameters: (1) total percent time pH less than 4.0, (2) percent time pH less than 4.0 in the upright period, (3) percent time pH less than 4.0 in the recumbent period, (4) the total number of reflux episodes, (5) the total number of reflux episodes longer than 5 minutes, and (6) the duration of the longest reflux episode over a 24-hour span of time.[16] From multiple physiologic studies of acid clearance it is evident that the acid clearance time in normal individuals is longer during sleep than during periods of wakefulness. Similarly, patients with GERD and nighttime symptoms experience greater acid exposure times when compared to daytime reflux patients.[17] Using simultaneous monitoring of esophageal pH and polysomnography, a recent study was conducted in 81 patients with sleep disturbance and heartburn and 39 controls with neither sleep problems nor heartburn. This study showed no difference in reflux event (27% versus 33%), but acid exposure time was longer in patients with sleep disturbances than in the control group (9.5% versus 1.6%; $P < 0.05$).[18] Nocturnal or sleep-related acid reflux therefore has the potential to be more harmful than daytime or upright reflux due to extended acid exposure time.

The relationship between an arousal or awakening and a reflux event is quite complex. Poh et al evaluated 39 patients with heartburn and/or regurgitation and 9 healthy controls and examined the association between conscious awakenings and acid reflux.[19] Of the GERD patients, 71.4% had conscious awakenings associated with acid reflux as compared to none in the control group. Similarly, 51.9% of conscious awakenings were associated with a reflux event in the GERD group and none of the awakenings were associated with an event in the control group. The number of awakenings was statistically significantly higher in the GERD group. Interestingly, 85.6% of conscious awakenings precede the reflux event. In a study from Freidin et al, patients with erosive esophagitis were evaluated using pH, manometry, and polysomnography. All but one reflux event was noted to occur during stage II of sleep in the GERD group. However, this was also the stage in which most patients spent the most amount of time. When the tracings were further analyzed, it was observed that there was an arousal 5 to 10 seconds prior to the reflux event.[20] These conscious awakenings may interrupt sleep; a high arousal index has been shown to be associated with poor quality of sleep. These studies emphasize the complex relationship between sleep and reflux. Sleep disturbance in an otherwise asymptomatic individual may itself lead to reflux events.

In addition to sleep disturbances triggering a reflux event, sleep deprivation also appears to be an independent factor in the exacerbation of GERD symptoms. In a crossover study evaluating sleep deprivation and perception in the esophagus, Schey et al studied 10 patients with reflux esophagitis and 10 healthy controls. After sleep deprivation, the GERD patients had a significant decrease in lag time to report symptoms, an increase in intensity rating, and an increase in acid perfusion sensitivity as compared to nights of good sleep.[11] This effect may create a detrimental cycle in GERD patients. The cycle may exist in which a GERD event creates an arousal. The arousal promotes sleep deprivation. The sleep deprivation in turn exacerbates the esophageal sensitivity to acid reflux. Breaking this cycle becomes extremely important so as to prevent esophageal damage and to create a well-rested, productive patient.

In regard to the timing of acid reflux events, they appear to occur more frequently in the first half of sleep or in the first half of the patient being in the supine position as determined by pH analysis.[21,22] More specifically, the events occurred most often in the first 2 hours of sleep and declined in 2-hour intervals over the course of the evening.[23] This observation was evident in patients with erosive esophagitis, Barrett's esophagus, and in those with nonerosive esophagitis. The group of patients in which prolonged nocturnal acid reflux is most worrisome is those who already have significant reflux damage to the esophagus (eg, as in those with Barrett's esophagus). When specifically studying patients with Barrett's esophagus, they were noted to have significantly longer esophageal acid exposure times as a result of more episodes of acid reflux during sleep.[24]

It has been proposed that *nocturnal heartburn* be defined as reflux symptoms associated with sleep disturbance, nocturnal arousal, and early morning awakening.[25] However, in addition to disturbed sleep in GERD patients, our group, Orr, and others have studied patients with complaints of sleep disturbance (without heartburn symptoms) who had simultaneous pH monitoring and polysomnography.[7,26] As a result, patients with disturbed sleep were not noted to have more reflux, but did have significantly prolonged acid exposure as compared to the healthy controls.[26] These studies suggests that the duration of acid exposure is an important factor in causing not just sleep disturbance but reflux events as well. Only a few studies have objectively evaluated the sleep parameters of patients without heartburn symptoms but who experience sleep disturbance.[27] Using objective analysis, it has been suggested that in perhaps 25% to 35% of patients with disturbed sleep, without known GERD or daytime heartburn symptoms, the etiology of the sleep disturbance may be gastroesophageal acid reflux.[7,27] From these data there appears to be a subset of patients who are experiencing sleep disturbance without overt reflux symptoms, termed the *silent nocturnal reflux group*. This prolonged and unrecognized acid exposure puts these patients at risk for esophageal complications, disturbed sleep, and absenteeism at work.

Recent advances in our ability to measure duodenogastroesophageal reflux have increased our knowledge on the importance of this nonacid component of the refluxate in the pathogenesis of GERD. The body of data that is accumulating indicates that nonacid reflux, in particular duodenogastroesophageal reflux, does not appear to cause significant damage to the esophageal mucosa on its own; however, in combination with acid, it can have deleterious effects.[28] Multichannel intraluminal impedance with pH monitoring is a highly sensitive method for the detection of all types of gastroesophageal refluxate and allows classification of reflux episodes as acid or nonacid.[29] In a study of 100 patients receiving twice-daily PPI therapy who underwent impedance/pH monitoring, it was found that this patient group had a significantly higher number of nonacid reflux episodes in the recumbent position.[30] Although the importance of duodenogastroesophageal reflux is still unknown, it is being increasingly acknowledged in light of the growing evidence that it plays an important role in the pathogenesis of GERD and possibly sleep disturbance.

THE CLINICAL IMPORTANCE OF GERD-RELATED SLEEP DISTURBANCE

As discussed earlier in this chapter, nocturnal reflux and its associated sleep arousal response have been implicated in sleep disruption and poor daytime performance/productivity. *Insomnia* is defined as difficulty in initiating or maintaining sleep and/or the sensation of nonrestorative sleep in the context of adequate opportunity to sleep, associated with the impairments of daytime functioning.[31] Insomnia is a common complaint that affects 30% of the population in the United States and more than 50% of the population over age 65. In an attempt to attain more restful sleep, many individuals seek sleep aids. Sleep aids, which include prescribed and over-the-counter medications, are commonly utilized by insomnia sufferers with an estimated 15% of the US population reporting their use.[32-34] Some medications used to manage sleep disturbances may aggravate GERD. For example, in an epidemiologic study, benzodiazepines have been shown to be significantly associated with heartburn during sleep.[9] In both animal models and humans, benzodiazepines decreased basal lower esophageal sphincter pressure and increased the numbers of GERD events.[35] Nonbenzodiazepine hypnotics include zolpidem, which binds to gamma-aminobutyric acid-A receptors, facilitating sleep onset and reducing the arousal threshold. Little information is available regarding the impact of hypnotic medications on arousals during sleep. However, research has been suggestive that hypnotic medications suppress nocturnal arousals, leading to prolonged acid exposure and mucosal injury over time.[36]

In a study from our group in 2009, patients with and without GERD were administered zolpidem and underwent simultaneous esophageal pH recording and standard polysomnography. Nocturnal acid exposure resulted in sleep arousal 89% of the time in participants (with and without GERD) who were given a placebo, but only 40% in those given zolpidem. In patients with GERD given zolpidem, acid reflux events lasted an average of 63.06 seconds when no arousal occurred and an average of 49.2 seconds when an arousal was recorded.[36] In a subgroup of insomnia patients with silent GERD, hypnotic medication use without acid-suppressive treatment may be especially damaging because acid exposure lasts longer and places the esophagus at risk for complications (eg, esophagitis, Barrett's esophagus, and adenocarcinoma). Patients who are awakened by nocturnal GERD events are able to mount defenses, including the usage of antireflux therapy, increased initiation of swallows, and increased peristalsis, whereas those patients who remain asleep during episodes may experience more mucosal injury.[37]

TREATMENT OF GERD-RELATED SLEEP DISTURBANCE

The cycle of GERD inducing poor sleep, which further aggravates GERD, may be interrupted by aggressive acid-reducing therapy. Several studies have evaluated the efficacy of PPI therapy for sleep disturbances in patients with GERD, but few randomized, blinded placebo-controlled clinical trials are available.[7,38-41] In a large study, Fass[37] showed that treatment with dexlansoprazole improved nocturnal heartburn and GERD-related sleep disturbances based on questionnaire analysis. Johnson and colleagues performed a large, multicenter randomized, double-blind, placebo-controlled trial utilizing esomeprazole (20 and 40 mg) or a placebo for 6 weeks in 675 adults with GERD-associated sleep disturbance. Fifty percent of the esomeprazole-treated subjects had resolution of nighttime heartburn, and by 4 weeks, 73% of the esomeprazole-treated subjects had resolution of their GERD-associated sleep disturbance. Both doses of esomeprazole resulted in improved sleep quality, a reduction in lost work hours, and increased work productivity.[38] In another study using rabeprazole for sleep-related GERD with 24-hour pH esophageal monitoring study with polysomnography, Orr et al observed that rabeprazole reduced overall acid reflux and improved subjective indices of sleep quality. However, this study failed to show any objective improvement of sleep parameters after acid suppression.[39] Ideally, PPIs for treatment of nocturnal GERD should provide rapid onset of action and symptom relief, as well as sustained action throughout the sleeping interval.

Although data are mounting, treating a sleep-disturbed patient (without GERD) with acid suppression alone has not been proven as of yet, and more data are needed. Data regarding other treatments for GERD (eg, fundoplication and its effect on sleep parameters) have been very limited. Eleven patients with heartburn undergoing fundoplication 8 to 10 weeks after surgery all reported an improvement of subjective sleep disturbances but not the objective sleep parameters.[42]

CONCLUSION

Sleep disturbance may be considered among the most important of the extraesophageal manifestations of GERD. Recent research has indicated that nighttime GERD symptoms are exceedingly common, occurring in nearly three-quarters of patients who report symptoms associated with reflux. Although nocturnal acid reflux can be asymptomatic, an astute clinician may notice poor sleep as a predictor of possible nocturnal GERD. In review of the basic mechanism, a reflux event triggers a sleep arousal, which in turn leads to swallow-induced esophageal acid clearance (Figure 5-2). This arousal-related sequence of events may lead to disturbed sleep, feelings of fatigue and daytime sleepiness, and a decrease in quality of life. PPIs have been shown to decrease gastroesophageal acid reflux and therefore are the main treatment option available for disturbed sleep due to GERD. A hypnotic medication such as zolpidem decreases the physiologic sleep arousal and thus increases nocturnal acid exposure by inhibiting the swallow reflex. This can lead to esophageal mucosa injury including erosive esophagitis, Barrett's esophagus, or even adenocarcinoma of the esophagus.

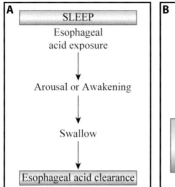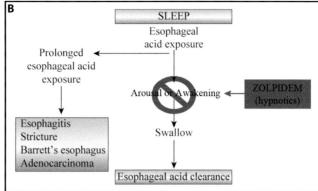

Figure 5-2. (A) A reflux event triggers a sleep arousal, which in turn leads to an arousal followed by swallow-induced esophageal acid clearance. (B) Hypnotic medication decreases the physiologic sleep arousal and thus increases noctural acid exposure by inhibiting the swallow reflex, which can lead to esophageal mucosa injury and possible Barrett's esophagus.

REFERENCES

1. The Gallup Organization. A Gallup survey on heartburn across America. Princeton, NJ: Author; 1988.
2. Shaker R, Castell DO, Schoenfeld PS, Spechler SJ. Nighttime heartburn is an under-appreciated clinical problem that impacts sleep and daytime function: the results of a Gallup survey conducted on behalf of the American Gastroenterological Association. *Am J Gastroenterol.* 2003;98:1487-1493.
3. Orr WC. Sleep and gastroesophageal reflux: what are the risks? *Am J Med.* 2003;115(suppl 3A):109S-113S.
4. Orr WC, Allen ML, Robinson M. The pattern of nocturnal and diurnal esophageal acid exposure in the pathogenesis of erosive mucosal damage. *Am J Gastroenterol.* 1994;89:509-512.
5. Locke G III, Talley NJ, Fert S, et al. Prevalence and clinical spectrum of gastroesophageal reflux: a population-based study in Olmsted County, Minnesota. *Gastroenterology.* 1997;112:1448-1456.
6. Farup C, Kleinman L, Sloan S, et al. The impact of nocturnal symptoms associated with gastroesophageal reflux disease on health-related quality of life. *Arch Intern Med.* 2001;161:45-52.
7. DiMarino AJ, Banwait KS, Echinger E, et al. The effect of gastro-oesophageal reflux and omeprazole on key sleep parameters. *Aliment Pharmacol Ther.* 2005;22:325-329.
8. Mody R, Bolge SC, Kannan H, Fass R. Effects of gastroesophageal reflux disease on sleep and outcomes. *Clin Gastroenterol Hepatol.* 2009;7:953-959.
9. Fass R, Quan SF, O'Connor GT, et al. Predictors of heartburn during sleep in a large prospective cohort study. *Chest.* 2005;127:1658-1666.
10. Jansson C, Nordenstedt H, Wallander MA, et al. A population-based study showing an association between gastroesophageal reflux disease and sleep problems. *Clin Gastroenterol Hepatol.* 2009;7:960-965.
11. Schey R, Dickman R, Parthasarathy S, et al. Sleep deprivation is hyperalgesic in patients with gastroesophageal reflux disease. *Gastroenterology.* 2007;133:1787-1795.
12. Zanation AM, Senior BA. The relationship between extraesophageal reflux (EER) and obstructive sleep apnea (OSA). *Sleep Med Rev.* 2005;9:453-458.
13. Orr WC, Robinson MG, Johnson LF. The effect of esophageal acid volume on arousals from sleep and acid clearance. *Chest.* 1991;99:351-354.
14. Orr WC, Robinson MG, Johnson LF. Acid clearance during sleep in the pathogenesis of reflux esophagitis. *Dig Dis Sci.* 1981;26:423-427.
15. Orr WC, Johnson LF. Response to different levels of esophageal acidification during waking and sleep. *Dig Dis Sci.* 1998;43:241-245.
16. Johnson LF, Demeester TR. Twenty-four-hour pH monitoring of the distal esophagus. A quantitative measure of gastroesophageal reflux. *Am J Gastroenterol.* 1974;62:325-332.
17. Orr WC, Eisenbruch S, Harnish MJ, et al. Proximal migration of esophageal acid perfusion during waking and sleep. *Am J Gastroenterol.* 2000;95:37-42.
18. Orr WC, Goodrich S, Fernstrom P, et al. Occurrence of nighttime gastroesophageal reflux in disturbed and normal sleepers. *Clin Gastroenterol Hepatol.* 2008;6:1099-1104.

19. Poh CH, Allen L, Gasiorowska A, et al. Conscious awakenings are commonly associated with acid reflux events in patients with gastroesophageal reflux disease. *Clin Gastroenterol Hepatol.* 2010;8:851-857.

20. Freidin N, Fisher MJ, Taylor W, et al. Sleep and nocturnal acid reflux in normal subjects and patients with reflux oesophagitis. *Gut.* 1991;32:1275-1279.

21. Dickman R, Green, Fass S, et al. Relationships between sleep quality and pH monitoring findings in persons with gastroesophageal reflux disease. *J Clin Sleep Med.* 2007;3:505-513.

22. Hila A, Castell DO. Nightime reflux is primarily an early event. *J Clin Gastroenterol.* 2005;39:579-583.

23. Dickman R, Parthasaranthy S, Malagon IB, et al. Comparison of the distribution of oesophageal acid exposure throughout the sleep period among the different gastro-oesophageal reflux disease groups. *Aliment Pharmacol Ther.* 2007;26:41-48.

24. Orr WC, Lackey C, Robinson MG, et al. Esophageal acid clearance during sleep in patients with Barrett's esophagus. *Dig Dis Sci.* 1988;33:654-659.

25. Gerson LB, Fass R. A systematic review of the definitions, prevalence, and response to treatment of nocturnal gastroesophageal reflux disease. *Clin Gastroenterol Hepatol.* 2009;7:372-378.

26. Orr WC, Goodrich S, Fernstrom P, et al. Occurrence of nighttime gastroesophageal reflux in disturbed and normal sleepers. *Clin Gastroenterol Hepatol.* 2008;6:1099-1104.

27. Shaheen NJ, Madanack RD, Alattar M, et al. Gastroesophageal reflux disease as an etiology of sleep disturbance in subjects with insomnia and minimal reflux symptoms: a pilot study of prevalence and response to therapy. *Dig Dis Sci.* 2008;53:1493-1499.

28. Vaezi MF, Richter JE. Synergism of acid and duodenogastroesophageal reflux in complicated Barrett's esophagus. *Surgery.* 1995;117:699-704.

29. Tutuian R, Vela M F, Shay SS, et al. Multichannel intraluminal impedance in oesophageal function testing and gastrooesophageal reflux monitoring. *J Clin Gastroenterol.* 2003;37:206-215.

30. Clayton SB, Rife CC, Singh ER, et al. Twice-daily proton pump inhibitor therapy does not decrease the frequency of reflux episodes during nocturnal recumbency in patients with refractory GERD: analysis of 200 patients using multichannel intraluminal impedance-pH testing. *Dis Esophagus.* 2012;25(8):682-686.

31. Morin CM. The nature of insomnia and the need to refine our diagnostic criteria. *Psychosom Med.* 2000;62(4):483-485.

32. Ohayon MM. Epidemiology of insomnia: what we know and what we still need to learn. *Sleep Med Review.* 2002;6:97.

33. Shochat T, Umphress J, Israel AG, et al. Insomnia in primary care patients. *Sleep.* 1999;22:(suppl 2):S359.

34. Morphy H, Dunn KM, Lewis M, et al. Epidemiology of insomnia: a longitudinal study in a UK population. *Sleep.* 2007;30:274.

35. Hall AW, Moossa AR, Clark J, Cooley GR, Skinner DB. The effects of premedication drugs on the lower oesophageal high pressure zone and reflux status of rhesus monkeys and man. *Gut.* 1975;16:347-352.

36. Gagliardi GS, Shah AP, Goldstein M, et al. Effect of zolpidem on the sleep arousal response to nocturnal esophageal acid exposure. *Clin Gastroenterol Hepatol.* 2009;9:948-952.

37. Fass R. The relationship between gastroesophageal reflux disease and sleep. *Curr Gastroenterol Rep.* 2009;11(3):202-208.

38. Johnson DA, Orr WC, Crawley JA, et al. Effect of esomeprazole on nighttime heartburn and sleep quality in patients with GERD: a randomized, placebo-controlled trial. *Am J Gastroenterol.* 2005;100:1914-1922.

39. Orr WC, Goodrich S, Robert J. The effect of acid suppression on sleep patterns and sleep-related gastro-oesophageal reflux. *Aliment Pharmacol Ther.* 2005;21:103-108.

40. Rackoff A, Agrawal A, Hila A, Mainie I, Tutuian R, Castell DO. Histamine-2 receptor antagonists at night improve gastroesophageal reflux disease symptoms for patients on proton pump inhibitor therapy. *Dis Esophagus.* 2005;18:370-373.

41. Fass R, Johnson DA, Orr WC, et al. The effect of dexlansoprazole MR on nocturnal heartburn and GERD-related sleep disturbances with symptomatic GERD. *Am J Gastroenterol.* 2011;106:421-431.

42. Cohen JA, Arain A, Harris PA, et al. Surgical trial investigating nocturnal gastroesophageal reflux and sleep (STINGERS). *Surg Endosc.* 2003;17:394-400.

chapter 6

GERD and Oral Manifestations

Mabi Singh, DMD, MS; Britta Magnuson, DMD; and
Athena Papas, DMD, PhD

Numerous studies have confirmed a significant association between gastroesophageal reflux disease (GERD) and involvement of the soft and hard tissue of the oral cavity in both adults and children. The signs and symptoms include dental erosion, halitosis, water brash (eg, sialorrhea, ptyalism), mouth sores (eg, mucosal ulceration), erythema of mucosa, taste disturbances, burning sensation, globus, dysphagia, odynophagia, and coughing. Dental erosion is the primary extraesophageal manifestation of GERD and will be discussed in detail in this chapter. Along with dental erosion, patients with GERD may also present with a higher incidence of canker sores, burning mouth sensation, sensitivity, and sour taste compared to a healthy population.[1-5]

There is a lack of understanding, adequate knowledge, and consensus among dentists and physicians alike, on typical and atypical manifestations of GERD in the oral cavity.

PROTECTIVE FACTORS AND THE ROLE OF SALIVA

Saliva is the most important biological factor that protects oral structures. The water content of the saliva dilutes the concentration of intrinsic and extrinsic acid introduced into the oral cavity and is primarily neutralized by the buffering capability of the salivary constituents (ie, water, bicarbonates, ammonia, urea, sialin, phosphates, and proteins).[6,7]

Saliva is also an important factor in the formation of acquired dental pellicle (ie, the selective binding salivary glycoproteins that deposit as an organic film on tooth surfaces).[8] The formation of dental pellicle creates a barrier and prevents direct exposure of the tooth surface to intrinsic and extrinsic acidic contents. Neurological stimuli triggered by acid in the oral cavity increases stimulated salivary production thereby increasing the buffering capacity (ie, bicarbonates), diluting and clearing acid from the mucosal and calcified surfaces, and maintaining homeostasis of the oral cavity. In stimulated saliva,

DiMarino AJ Jr, Cohen S, eds.
Extraesophageal Manifestations of GERD (pp 85-94).

bicarbonate buffers both the extrinsic and intrinsic acid, accounting for approximately 90% of the saliva buffer capacity.[9,10] As the stimulation increases, the concentration of bicarbonates also increases as does the volume of saliva, raising the pH from 6.6 in unstimulated saliva to 7.4 in stimulated saliva.[6,11-13] Consequently, the net result is that the stimulated saliva contains more bicarbonate than resting saliva. Thus, in a healthy individual, either extrinsic or intrinsic acid will maximally stimulate salivary flow and increase buffer capacity.[14,15] Also, a supersaturated concentration of calcium and phosphate in healthy saliva promotes remineralization of demineralized tooth surfaces.

The protective factors of saliva may be diminished in those with salivary hypofunction. Salivary hypofunction can be caused by a variety of conditions such as Sjögren's syndrome, rheumatoid arthritis, radiation to the head and neck region, and polypharmacy.

There are more than 450 medications that cause salivary hypofunction, a condition that affects an estimated 20% of adults worldwide. Additionally, many elderly patients are on multiple medications that affect salivary flow and adversely affect the oral cavity.

Dental erosion occurs when the rate of demineralization exceeds the rate of remineralization of the calcified dental tissue. The hydroxyapatite crystals in enamel dissolve at the critical pH level of 5.5 and in dentin at a level of 6.9. Medically compromised patients may have severely diminished or absent saliva, increasing the rate of progression of dental erosion. The new elderly are retaining their teeth longer, consequently increasing exposure of root surfaces composed of dentin as the gingival recedes, placing the more vulnerable root surface at risk of developing erosive lesions.[16] A study conducted by us at Tufts found erosion was high among 95 volunteers on xerogenic medication with 46% having evidence of erosion.[17]

Sjögren's syndrome is an autoimmune disease that causes severe xerostomia and xerophthalmia affecting primarily postmenopausal women as compared to men at a rate of 9:1. A survey conducted by the Sjögren's Syndrome Foundation in 2007 to 2008 of 1225 Sjögren's patients and 606 peer controls demonstrated that 49% of the patients with Sjögren's syndrome reported to have GERD compared to 19% of the peer controls.[18] Among 65 Sjögren's patients at Tufts University, 58% of those who reported GERD had erosive lesions and 41% of those who did not report GERD had lesions, suggesting that there is a high level of undiagnosed GERD in this population.[19]

EXTRAESOPHAGEAL SIGNS AND SYMPTOMS OF GERD

Sour (Bitter) Taste

Waking up with a sour (bitter) taste in the mouth is due to the accumulation of refluxate in the oral cavity during sleep when the circadian variation of the salivary flow is at the minimum and there is decreased oromotor activity.[20] Flushing or clearance of the liquid contents of refluxate is at the lowest, which results in a sour taste in the mouth upon waking. The severity may depend upon the amount and the pH of refluxate. The gastric acid produced by parietal cells in the stomach contains hydrochloric acid, potassium chloride, and sodium chloride.[21] Absence of stimulated saliva during sleep reduces the buffering capacity of the saliva as stimulated saliva is an effective buffer due to its high bicarbonate content.

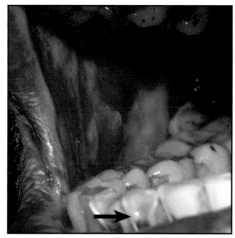

Figure 6-1. Mucosal irritation due to GERD and slush weighs on incisors.

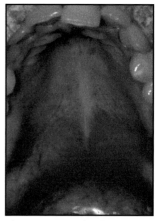

Figure 6-2. Palatal irritation due to GERD.

Halitosis

Research done by Moshkowitz et al found a strong association between halitosis and GERD. Among the possible correlation of halitosis and GERD, direct damage or injury of the oral mucosa may cause inflammation of the tissue.[22] Halitosis has also often been reported among the symptoms related to *Helicobacter pylori* infection and GERD.[23]

Sialorrhea (Water Brash or Ptyalism)

The acidic refluxate from the stomach causes gustatory stimulation of the salivary center in the medulla. Thus, neurophysiological stimulation of the salivary glands increases the salivary production to neutralize the stimulants. Excessive foamy, ropy mucus is reported and typically referred to as *water brash*. The resulting drooling of saliva and need for constant expectoration of salivary contents may become a social stigma.[24]

Mouth Sores (Mucosal Ulcerations) and Erythema of the Mucosa

While there are no pathognomonic mucosal lesions for GERD,[25] the direct exposure of low pH gastric refluxate to oral tissues may alter the oromucosal defense and necrotize and slough off the mucosa, creating a breakdown in the continuity of mucosal lining, which results in ulceration and inflammation. Mucosal tissues in the oral cavity vary in thickness and level of keratinization. Tissues with lower levels of keratinization are more vulnerable to acidic injury (Figures 6-1 through 6-3). One of the earlier signs of GERD may be the bilateral or unilateral erythema of the anterior pillars of tonsils, depending on the sleeping position.

Taste Disturbances and Chemosensory Changes

Our studies and others have found that patients suffering from GERD have higher significant risk of burning sensation (ie, glossodynia) of the oral cavity and xerostomia.[26] The low pH content of the refluxate may cause irritation of the highly innervated parts of the oral cavity translating into a burning sensation of the tongue.

Figure 6-3. Irritation of uvula and anterior tonsillar pillars.

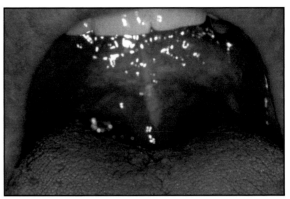

Figure 6-4. Loss of vertical height and coexisting carious lesions with erosion.

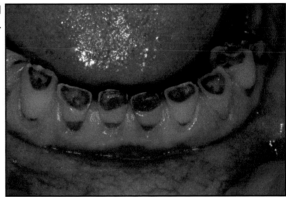

Dental Carious Lesions

Even though caries is primarily related to bacterial acid, dental carious lesions and tooth surface loss can coexist. The tooth surface loss, due to acidic challenges, exposes dentin of teeth, which is more susceptible to both bacterial and intrinsic factors (Figure 6-4).

Tooth Surface Loss

Tooth surface loss by erosion occurs due to acidity and the erosive potential in the oral cavity from intrinsic or extrinsic acid that has exceeded the buffering capability and neutralizing functions of normal saliva and salivary proteins. The term *corrosion* has also been used to describe tooth surface loss caused by chemical and electrochemical actions.[27] Dental erosion occurs when the rate of demineralization exceeds the rate of remineralization of the calcified dental tissue. The hydroxyapatite crystals in enamel dissolve at the critical pH level of 5.5 and in dentin at a level of 6.9. In a normal situation, tooth structure is remineralized with the formation of hydroxyfluoroapatite crystals, which are more resistant to acidic attacks. Frequent acid exposure increases the demineralization of tooth structures. Chronic regurgitation or reflux of gastric contents, including gastric acid with a pH well below 2, is a significant cause of the dental erosion.[28-30] Dental erosion can be considered an atypical manifestation of GERD. The association of GERD and dental erosion was first reported by Howden as a representing symptom in hiatus hernia.[31] Eighty-three percent of the patients with dental erosion had evidence of GERD.[6,32]

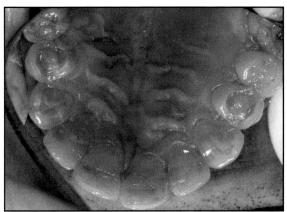

Figure 6-5. Cupping, pitting, and loss of cusps.

Due to loss of surface enamel and exposure of underlying dentin, erosion can cause the teeth to look yellowish. In cases of severe erosion, sensitivity and the loss of the vertical height of teeth, and consequently temporomandibular joint damage, can also be experienced. Other complications may include difficulty in eating and chewing with a threat to the pulp and integrity of the teeth. Thus, various effects on the functions, aesthetics, and overall quality of life can be compromised depending upon the severity of dental erosion. The cost to maintain and restore dentition may add an extra burden to the sufferers of GERD.

DIAGNOSIS OF TOOTH SURFACE LOSS DUE TO EROSION

Dental structure is a mineralized tissue that goes through a dynamic process of remineralization and demineralization in the oral cavity. Calcium and phosphate ions leech from the dental structure in the presence of acid and normal-functioning saliva, which is supersaturated with respect to calcium and phosphate. There is a reuptake of these ions in the presence of fluoride. In an adverse chemical environment (excluding bacterial plaque acid) or with chelators acting on plaque-free tooth surfaces, the irreversible loss of mineral components from dental tissue occurs through mineral dissolution and is known as *erosion*. Erosion does not have any direct association with mechanical or traumatic actions or with dental carious lesions produced by bacterial acid. However, dental erosion can often coexist with attrition (ie, tooth tissue loss caused by antagonistic tooth-to-tooth physical contact), abfraction (ie, physical wear as a result of tensile or sheer stress usually at the cemento-enamel region), and abrasion (ie, physical wear caused by mechanical processes involving foreign abrasive substances). As a result, the encompassment of various types of dental lesions may make the differentiation of erosion quite difficult to assess.

The pattern of tooth wear due to erosion will differ according to the severity of etiological factors. Damage to the tooth structures because of the GERD may be very characteristic and include wear on the occlusal (chewing) surfaces of molars (Figure 6-5). Because of acidic challenges in the oral cavity, the tooth surface loss of the occlusal surface, especially on the cusp tips, can result in saucer-shaped cupping (Figure 6-6) and flattening of the whole occlusal surface. If the occlusal surfaces contain metallic restorations, a restoration may appear to be shiny due to acid etching and protrude from the tooth surface. This is called the *proud restoration* (Figure 6-7). Erosion can vary from minor and subtle changes on the incisal surface to generalized thinning of enamel and exposure of underlying dentin (Figure 6-8).

Figure 6-6. Cupping on the occlusal surface of a tooth and exposure of dentin.

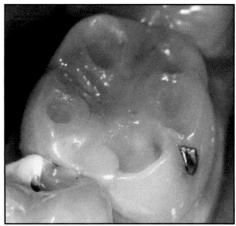

Figure 6-7. Loss of surrounding tooth surface leading to the appearance of restorations protruding out of the teeth. Note the shiny appearance of metallic restoration due to etching of acid.

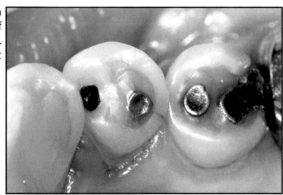

Figure 6-8. Initial thinning of enamel and increased translucency on upper incisors.

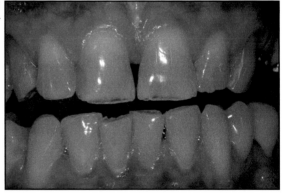

When the erosive lesions occur at the buccal surfaces of the teeth, the width of the lesions is characteristically greater than the depth in contrast to abrasion (eg, toothpaste abrasion), in which the depth may be greater and typically has a "V" shape. Therefore, the erosive lesions form concavities at the cervical area (ie, along the gum line) and the preservation of enamel "cuff" in gingival crevice is often seen (Figure 6-9). In severe cases, pulp exposure may occur, especially in the palatal molar area (Figure 6-10).

Incisal edges, palatal surfaces of the maxillary teeth, and occlusal surfaces of the mandibular posterior teeth are affected by GERD (see Figure 6-9). The labial and facial surfaces

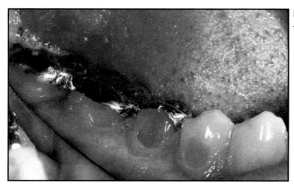

Figure 6-9. Loss of tooth surface due to acid on buccal surfaces.

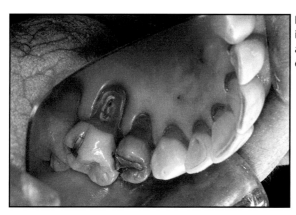

Figure 6-10. Recession of gum exposing the root surfaces, which are readily abraded and eroded, leading to pulpal exposure.

of the maxillary teeth and the buccal and occlusal surfaces of the mandibular teeth are affected due to the exposure of extrinsic acids.

The prevalence of dental erosion is on the rise both in children[33] and adults. In a systemic review, Pace et al showed a strong association between GERD and dental erosion.[3] The severity of dental erosion is correlated in the presence of GERD symptoms. Although these studies differed in design, GERD diagnostic methods, duration, and follow-up, the median prevalence of dental erosion in GERD patients was 24% (range: 5% to 47%) and the median prevalence of GERD in dental erosion patients was 32.5% (range: 21% to 83%). The median prevalence of dental erosion in the pediatric population was 17% with a large range of 14% to 87%.[3] Significant associations were also found between erosion and diagnosed reflux disease (odds ratio 2.772; $p \geq 0.005$) in a group of 249 Icelanders.[28] According to Milosevic, the evidence used in the review was plausible, but the strength of the association and the epidemiological evidence was unclear.[34]

MANAGEMENT

To date, no evidence-based guidelines or studies exist for the prevention or treatment of GERD-related dental erosion. When diagnosed with GERD, physicians should routinely refer their patients to a dental professional for assessment, definitive treatment, and to provide appropriate preventive protocols to ensure control and limit further damage of the soft and hard tissue of the oral cavity. Alternately, if the typical (and atypical) patterns of GERD are present, dentists should refer their patients to a physician for a definitive diagnosis and medical intervention of GERD. Early recognition, diagnosis, and management of GERD are key factors for successful treatment of extraesophageal lesions and dental erosion.

Increasing Salivary Flow

GERD patients may also suffer from xerostomia. Since saliva is the most important biological factor that prevents erosion, measures should be taken to increase salivary flow. Cholinergic agents such as sialogogues (eg, pilocarpine HCl and cevimeline HCl) have been shown to improve salivary flow and provide the needed protective actions. However, these cholinergic agents may also promote gastric acid production so titration of doses and caution should be observed. These medications should be taken along with food. Salivary flow can also be increased by mechanical and gustatory stimulation (eg, chewing sugar-free xylitol gum or using a power toothbrush on the tongue to stimulate saliva).

Controlling the Acidic Environment

It is important to address the acidic environment of the oral cavity to manage GERD-related signs and symptoms. To reduce quantitative acid and neutralize acidic concentration in the oral cavity, it is advisable to rinse with water, milk, sodium bicarbonate (baking soda in water; pH 8), or low fluoride-containing rinse. It is also advisable to use pH-elevating oral sprays, brush with fluoride-containing amorphous calcium phosphate (ACP) toothpaste, and apply casein phosphopeptide-based calcium and phosphate (CPP-ACP). It is important to note that immediately brushing after the consumption of acidic drinks or foods should be discouraged because due to the decreased microhardness of the enamel and dentine, the tooth structure may be abraded away easily. Consumption of neutralizing foods (eg, cheese and dairy products) may also help to control the acidic environment.

Remineralizing the Tooth Structure

Every attempt should be made to remineralize erosive lesions and to stop the progression of erosion. Fluoride helps with the reuptake of available calcium and phosphate present in saliva. Fluorides are available in various concentrations and can be applied by the patients (eg, sodium fluoride [5000 ppm] toothpaste) or professionally via varnishes (26,000 ppm of fluoride) without the need of any specific procedure. The reuptake of minerals can be enhanced by supplying or applying ions of calcium and phosphate in various forms These include ACP-soluble calcium and phosphate ions in the form of rinses, CPP-ACP, and calcium sodium phosphosilicate, a nanosized, bioactive glass.

Restoration of Teeth

Tooth restoration depends upon individual considerations, needs, and the degree of damage. The control of the acidic regurgitation of GERD must be confirmed to initiate more complicated and definitive dental treatments to ensure success. As temporary or transient restorations, resin-based composites and glass ionomer cements can be used. The restorative procedures range from simple restorations with reproduction of anatomical forms to onlays, veneers, and full-mouth rehabilitation with ceramic crowns.

CONCLUSION

When a diagnosis of GERD is suspected or established, physicians should refer their patients to a dental professional for a definitive diagnosis and preventive treatment plan to stop the progression of dental erosion and other oral manifestations involving soft tissue. It is also recommended that when a dental professional finds typical or atypical dental erosion and other oral manifestations involving soft tissue, the dentist should urge the patient to seek evaluation and assessment of possible GERD from a physician. Early recognition, diagnosis, and management of GERD are key factors for successful treatment of dental erosion and other extraesophageal and oral manifestations.

REFERENCES

1. Ranjitkar S, Smales RJ, Kaidonis JA. Oral manifestations of gastroesophageal reflux disease. *J Gastroenterol Hepatol*. 2012;27(1):21-27.
2. Di Fede O, Di Liberto C, Occhipinti G, et al. Oral manifestations in patients with gastro-oesophageal reflux disease: a single-center case-control study. *J Oral Pathol Med*. 2008;37(6):336-340.
3. Pace F, Pallotta S, Tonini M, Vakil N, Bianchi Porro G. Systematic review: gastro-oesophageal reflux disease and dental lesions. *Aliment Pharmacol Ther*. 2008;27(12):1179-1186.
4. Heidelbaugh JJ, Gill AS, Van Harrison R, Nostrant TT. Atypical presentations of gastroesophageal reflux disease. *Am Fam Physician*. 2008;78(4):483-488.
5. Fass R, Achem SR, Harding S, Mittal RK, Quigley E. Review article: supra-oesophageal manifestations of gastro-oesophageal reflux disease and the role of night-time gastro-oesophageal reflux. *Aliment Pharmacol Ther*. 2004;(20 suppl 9):26-38.
6. Bardow A, Madsen J, Nauntofte B. The bicarbonate concentration in human saliva does not exceed the plasma level under normal physiological conditions. *Clin Oral Investig*. 2000;4(4):245-253.
7. Dawes C, Chebib FS. The influence of previous stimulation and the day of the week on the concentrations of protein and the main electrolytes in human parotid saliva. *Arch Oral Biol*. 1972;17(9):1289-1301.
8. Hara AT, Ando M, Gonzalez-Cabezas C, Cury JA, Serra MC, Zero DT. Protective effect of the dental pellicle against erosive challenges in situ. *J Dent Res*. 2006;85(7):612-616.
9. Pedersen AM, Bardow A, Jensen SB, Nauntofte B. Saliva and gastrointestinal functions of taste, mastication, swallowing, and digestion. *Oral Dis*. 2002;8(3):117-129.
10. Park K, Hurley PT, Roussa E, et al. Expression of a sodium bicarbonate cotransporter in human parotid salivary glands. *Arch Oral Biol*. 2002;47(1):1-9.
11. Fenoll-Palomares C, Munoz Montagud JV, Sanchiz V, et al. Unstimulated salivary flow rate, pH and buffer capacity of saliva in healthy volunteers. *Rev Esp Enferm Dig*. 2004;96(11):773-783.
12. Moritsuka M, Kitasako Y, Burrow MF, Ikeda M, Tagami J, Nomura S. Quantitative assessment for stimulated saliva flow rate and buffering capacity in relation to different ages. *J Dent*. 2006;34(9):716-720.
13. Brand HS, Ligtenberg AJ, Bots CP, Nieuw Amerongen AV. Secretion rate and buffer capacity of whole saliva depend on the weight of the mechanical stimulus. *Int J Dent Hyg*. 2004;2(3):137-138.
14. Tschoppe P, Wolgin M, Pischon N, Kielbassa AM. Etiologic factors of hyposalivation and consequences for oral health. *Quintessence Int*. 2010;41(4):321-333.
15. Almstahl A, Wikstrom M. Electrolytes in stimulated whole saliva in individuals with hyposalivation of different origins. *Arch Oral Biol*. 2003;48(5):337-344.
16. Lussi A, Jaeggi T. Erosion—diagnosis and risk factors. *Clin Oral Investig*. 2008;(12 suppl 1):S5-S13.
17. Singh ML, Papas AS, Tzavaras E, Walanski AA, Barker ML, Gerlach RW. Clinical evaluation of erosion prevalence in a xerostomic population. International Association of Dental Research Conference. Vol Abstract #772. Miami, FL. 2009.
18. Sjögren's Syndrome Foundation. *Burden of Illness and General Health-Related Quality of Life in a U.S. Sjögren's Syndrome Population*. Bethesda, MD: Author; 2007.
19. Brown AA, Singh, ML, Papas AS. GERD, sialometry, and dental erosion in a Sjögren's syndrome population. International Association of Dental Research Conference. Vol Abstract #1348. San Diego, CA. 2011.
20. Dawes C. Circadian rhythms in human salivary flow rate and composition. *J Physiol*. 1972;220(3):529-545.
21. Yao X, Forte JG. Cell biology of acid secretion by the parietal cell. *Ann Rev Physiol*. 2003;65:103-131.
22. Moshkowitz M, Horowitz N, Leshno M, Halpern Z. Halitosis and gastroesophageal reflux disease: a possible association. *Oral Dis*. 2007;13(6):581-585.
23. Kinberg S, Stein M, Zion N, Shaoul R. The gastrointestinal aspects of halitosis. *Can J Gastroenterol*. 2010;24(9):552-556.
24. Boyce HW, Bakheet MR. Sialorrhea: a review of a vexing, a often unrecognized sign of oropharyngeal and esophageal disease. *J Clin Gastroenterol*. 2005;39(2):89-97.
25. Alfaro EV, Aps JK, Martens LC. Oral implications in children with gastroesophageal reflux disease. *Curr Opin Pediatr*. 2008;20(5):576-583.
26. Campisi G, Lo Russo L, Di Liberto C, et al. Saliva variations in gastro-oesophageal reflux disease. *J Dent*. 2008;36(4):268-271.

27. Grippo JO. Biocorrosion vs erosion: the 21st century and a time to change. *Compend Contin Educ Dent.* 2012;33(2):e33-e37.

28. Holbrook WP, Furuholm J, Gudmundsson K, Theodors A, Meurman JH. Gastric reflux is a significant causative factor of tooth erosion. *J Dent Res.* 2009;88(5):422-426.

29. Jarvinen V, Meurman JH, Hyvarinen H, Rytomaa I, Murtomaa H. Dental erosion and upper gastrointestinal disorders. *Oral Surg Oral Med Oral Pathol.* 1988;65(3):298-303.

30. Meurman JH, Toskala J, Nuutinen P, Klemetti E. Oral and dental manifestations in gastroesophageal reflux disease. *Oral Surg Oral Med Oral Pathol.* 1994;78(5):583-589.

31. Howden GF. Erosion as the presenting symptom in hiatus hernia. A case report. *Br Dent J.* 1971;131(10):455-456.

32. Schroeder PL, Filler SJ, Ramirez B, Lazarchik DA, Vaezi MF, Richter JE. Dental erosion and acid reflux disease. *Ann Intern Med.* 1995;122(11):809-815.

33. Nunn JH, Gordon PH, Morris AJ, Pine CM, Walker A. Dental erosion—changing prevalence? A review of British national childrens' surveys. *Int J Paediatr Dent.* 2003;13(2):98-105.

34. Milosevic A. Eating disorders and the dentist. *Br Dent J.* 1999;186(3):109-113.

Extraesophageal Manifestations in the Pediatric Population

Joan S. Di Palma, MD; Sheeja K. Abraham, MD; and
Rebecca O. Ramirez, MD, FAAP

Gastroesophageal reflux (GER) and gastroesophageal reflux disease (GERD) are among the most common issues addressed by pediatric gastroenterologists. All ages are affected, from the premature infant to the adolescent and young adult. However, the characteristics of GER vary the most in infants, who experience more frequent regurgitation and vomiting. Studies suggest that 3% to 10% of infants born prematurely (ie, birth weight < 1500 g) have GER.[1] Fifty percent of 2-month-old infants regurgitate 2 times a day. At 1 year of age, only 1% of infants regurgitate 2 times a day. The prevalence of GER symptoms in children 3 to 18 years of age is 1.8% to 2.2%.[2]

Transient lower esophageal sphincter relaxation (TLESR) is thought to be the major mechanism responsible for GER in adults and children.[3] However, there are additional physiological factors that contribute to GER in infants. Infants ingest twice the volume of liquids per day per kilogram of body weight as compared to adults (100 to 150 mL/kg/day versus 30 to 50 mL/kg/day). The volume of an infant's stomach is much smaller than an adult's stomach; therefore, the infant's stomach is more prone to distension, which can lead to an increase in TLESR.[4] Infants have a shorter intra-abdominal esophagus and a smaller acute angle of His than adults. The length of the lower esophageal sphincter (LES) in adults is 3 to 6 cm, compared to just a few millimeters in infants. These factors contribute to the weakening of the antireflux barrier.[4,5] The LES pressure is decreased in premature and term infants compared to adults (3.8 mm Hg in infants with < 29 weeks gestation, 18 mm Hg in term infants, and 20 to 40 mm Hg in adults).[1] Esophageal clearance is part of the "line of defense" against acid reflux. Swallowing saliva enhances peristalsis of the esophagus and helps to neutralize the refluxate. Infants have an increased number of nonpropagating esophageal contractions.[6] Swallowing decreases markedly during sleep. Adults swallow approximately 600 times during the day and approximately 50 times during sleep.[5] Infants spend a greater proportion of their day sleeping and are therefore less efficient at esophageal clearance for a greater part of their day. Infants are more prone to delayed

DiMarino AJ Jr, Cohen S, eds.
Extraesophageal Manifestations of GERD (pp 97-110).
© 2013 Taylor & Francis Group.

Table 7-1	Presenting Symptoms of GERD in Infants, Older Children, and Adolescents
INFANTS	**OLDER CHILDREN/ADOLESCENTS**
Persistent vomiting	Heartburn, painful burping
Feeding difficulties	Nausea
Poor weight gain	Epigastric abdominal pain
Irritability/arching	Dental erosions
Apnea/apparent life-threatening events	Cough, wheezing, hoarseness

gastric emptying, which increases intragastric pressure and TLESR.[4,7] Recently, there has been interest in a possible genetic basis for GERD. There has been concordance of GERD symptoms described in monozygotic twins. Family clustering of Barrett's esophagus and erosive esophagitis has been reported.[7]

Understandably, infants and children with underlying physical disorders will be more predisposed to GERD. These include congenital abnormalities of the gastrointestinal tract, such as diaphragmatic hernia, esophageal atresia, gastroschisis and omphalocele, hiatal hernia, and malrotation. Neurodevelopmental delay, physical stress, and infection can also exacerbate GER/GERD. The variety of age groups represented in the pediatric population naturally leads to a variability in GER/GERD presenting symptoms. Table 7-1 illustrates the difference between presenting symptoms of GER/GERD in infants, older children, and adolescents. Extraesophageal symptoms attributed to GER/GERD have been cited at all age ranges and include apnea/apparent life-threatening events (ALTE), respiratory symptoms, otitis media and sinusitis, feeding difficulties and irritability, and failure to thrive.

Until a child is 8 to 12 years of age, it is difficult to rely on verbalization of symptoms. Therefore, it is difficult to make a clinical diagnosis of GER/GERD in an infant based on symptoms alone. Vomiting suggests GER/GERD, but the differential diagnosis of vomiting in an infant or toddler is broad. Care must be taken to consider and exclude other causes of vomiting in this age group. Excellent references are available for this purpose.[4,8,9] There are several diagnostic modalities available to assist in making a diagnosis of GER/GERD. These include contrast radiography (barium esophagram or upper GI series), nuclear scintigraphy, 24-hour pH monitoring and 24-hour pH monitoring combined with multiple channel intraluminal impedance monitoring (MII), and endoscopy with biopsy. Analysis of fluid from the esophagus, upper respiratory tract, ear effusions for lipid-laden macrophages (LAM), pepsin, and bilirubin has also been proposed. Finally, empiric medical therapy for GERD symptoms is sometimes utilized as a diagnostic test.

Although a barium esophagram and upper GI series are excellent studies to evaluate anatomy, they are poor screens for GER/GERD. Because the duration of the test is brief, GER is frequently missed. The significance of visualized GER during the study is hard to interpret, because the GER may be physiological.[4,7] Nuclear scintigraphy is done by labeling milk or infant formula with technetium-99. The ingested bolus is followed for 1 hour. GER (acid and nonacid) can be identified, as well as pulmonary aspiration. Gastric emptying is also assessed. Limitations of the study are that evaluation standards are poorly established and that only immediate postprandial reflux is assessed. Pulmonary aspiration is rarely identified. Nuclear scintigraphy is generally not recommended for the evaluation of GER/GERD in infants and is rarely utilized in older children and adolescents.[4,7,8] Esophageal manometry is more helpful in explaining pathophysiology of GER/GERD than in diagnosis. Therefore, it is rarely performed solely to diagnose GER in a child.[4,5,7,10]

Endoscopy and esophageal biopsy are helpful at identifying complications of GERD, such as reflux esophagitis, esophageal strictures, and Barrett's esophagus. Esophageal biopsy is important because there is only a 50% correlation between the gross appearance of the esophagus and histologic findings. A normal esophagus does not exclude GER.[7,11,12] Visible breaks in the esophageal mucosa, esophageal ulcerations and erosions, and esophageal strictures are all highly suggestive of GERD. A full esophagogastroduodenoscopy is helpful at excluding entities other than GER that relate to symptoms (eg, eosinophilic esophagitis, infectious esophagitis, pill esophagitis, and inflammatory bowel disease).

Twenty-four-hour pH monitoring, either with standard antimony electrodes or with wireless pH monitoring (Bravo capsule, Given Imaging, Yoqneam, Israel), has been performed for many years. There is good reproducibility in the data for both methods.[13,14] There have been normal values established, and temporal associations between symptoms and GER can be made.[14-19] The interpretation of pH monitoring in premature infants is difficult. These infants feed frequently or are fed continuously via nasogastric tubes. Gastric pH is elevated by the presence of persistent breast milk or formula. Therefore, pH less than 4 is not seen as frequently during GER episodes. Assessing GER in the proximal esophagus is difficult, because saliva neutralizes the refluxate. Twenty-four-hour pH monitoring is currently not accepted as a valid means of evaluating GER in suspected extraesophageal reflux disease.[7]

MII in infants and children has been evaluated in comparison to and in concordance with 24-hour pH monitoring. The combined technique (24-hour pH-MII) identifies nonacid and weakly acid events, as well as acid events.[20,21] Correlation between symptoms is enhanced, even in premature infants.[22-26] Data from the German Pediatric Impedance Group, in 700 pediatric patients with gastrointestinal, neurological, and pulmonary symptoms, suggested that 45% of patients with GER would not have had GER detected without combined MII and pH monitoring.[27] The same study suggests that patients with extraesophageal symptoms of GER were more likely to have nonacid reflux events. Because pH-MII monitoring increases the accuracy of detecting all reflux events and correlates GER to symptoms, clinical decision making is enhanced.[28]

Although pH-MII monitoring has been a helpful addition in the process of diagnosing GER, the procedure is not without limitations. pH-MII monitoring is not helpful in predicting which patients have esophageal mucosal injury and reflux esophagitis.[29,30] Evaluating an MII tracing is difficult, and there are no established "normals" for all age groups.[7] There is considerable intraobserver variability in evaluating MII studies. Loots et al described a 42% correlation between experts' evaluations of MII and pH tracings. The authors suggest that automated analysis may be preferable at this time.[30]

Finally, diagnosis of GER by indirect means has been proposed for many years. The identification of LAM in bronchiolar secretions was proposed as suggestive of GER by Nussbaum et al in 1987.[31] In this study, 85% of patients with respiratory symptoms and positive testing for GER had LAM identified in bronchiolar secretions. Only 19% of patients with respiratory symptoms and no positive diagnostic tests for GER were positive for LAM. Rosen et al subsequently compared LAM to 24-hour pH studies and found no significant correlation between LAM and acid reflux identified on 24-hour pH probe or reflux esophagitis identified on esophageal biopsy.[32] The identification of pepsin in bronchiolar secretions and in middle ear effusions has suggested that pepsin may be of diagnostic utility in determining the cause of chronic respiratory symptoms and otitis media.[33-36] Further studies in this area are ongoing. There are few controlled studies that document that pepsin is not present in respiratory secretions and ear effusions in individuals without respiratory disease, GER, or recurrent otitis media.

The seriousness and impact of presenting symptoms dictate need for extensive diagnostic testing for GER. Once GER is documented, it is important to be able to relate GER temporally and/or causally to symptoms. In this way, a therapeutic plan can be devised. In this chapter, proposed extraesophageal complications of GER will be discussed. These include apnea and ALTE, excessive irritability and growth problems, and respiratory and ear, nose, and throat (ENT) symptoms.

APNEA AND APPARENT LIFE-THREATENING EVENTS

Apnea and ALTE occur primarily in infants less than 8 months old. They are among the most alarming and frightening occurrences to parents, caretakers, and physicians. ALTE consist of a variable combination of symptoms including apnea, respiratory symptoms (eg, cough, gagging, and choking), limpness or excessive irritability, and color change (eg, pallor, plethora, or cyanosis).[37] At times, the infant recovers spontaneously. At other times, the infant requires various interventions, such as stimulation or suctioning. The observer interprets the seriousness of the event and symptoms. In hospitalized premature infants, ALTE are detected by monitors and are reported by caretakers. ALTE events in premature infants can include bradycardia and oxygen desaturation. There is no clear evidence that ALTE leads to sudden infant death syndrome (SIDS), but there are rare case reports of SIDS in infants who have had ALTE episodes.[37-40]

Understandably, there has been a great deal of interest in defining the cause of ALTE in an infant. There are a variety of physical issues that can be implicated, including infection, metabolic or neurological disorders, cardiac disease, and child abuse.[7] GER was first implicated as a potential cause of ALTE more than 30 years ago.[41,42] Since that time, there have been several studies attempting to link ALTE and GER temporally. The evidence supporting the relationship between GER and ALTE is conflicting secondarily to the variable presentations and descriptions of the ALTE events and to the variety of diagnostic modalities for GER.[7] Many of the earlier studies utilized 24-hour pH monitoring, while more recent studies use 24-hour pH-MII.

Awake apnea has been temporally associated with GER.[43] This type of apnea is associated with airway obstruction and may not be pathologic, but may be an expression of a normal protective reflex stimulated by regurgitated gastric fluid or an inefficient swallow.[7] Utilizing combined pH monitoring and polysonography, a temporal relationship between apnea and GER during sleep and in the postprandial period can be identified.[39,44,45] However, Newman et al found a similar incidence of GER in control patients without ALTE.[44] Kahn et al, utilizing 24-hour pH monitoring of the proximal esophagus, found no temporal relationship between acid GER and apnea and bradycardia.[45] Both Paton et al and Walsh et al found no temporal relationship between acid GER and obstructive or central apnea.[46,47] More recent studies attempting to correlate GER and apnea have utilized MII in addition to pH monitoring and pneumogram. These studies can correlate acid, weakly acid, and nonacid GER events with ALTE. Unfortunately, the results are not consistent when studies are compared. Wenzl et al correlated 39% of 165 apneic episodes in 22 infants with acid and nonacid GER. Approximately 20% of the episodes were correlated with acid reflux and 9% were correlated with nonacid reflux.[48] Mousa et al linked only 15% of 527 apneic episodes to acid and nonacid GER.[49] Premature infants are at risk for concerning episodes of apnea and bradycardia. Using MII, Magistà et al identified an increase in weakly acidic GER in prematures.[50] Therefore, MII is potentially an important diagnostic tool for GER in premature infants. Peter et al studied 19 premature infants with combined pneumograms, pH, and MII. There were 2039 episodes of apnea, 188 episodes of desaturation, and 44 episodes of bradycardia observed. There were also 524 reflux events observed during the

6-hour recording. There was no significant correlation noted between apnea, bradycardia, desaturation, and reflux events.[51]

There are other factors that confuse the relationship between GER and ALTE. Studies have shown that SIDS is rare when infants are maintained in a supine position while sleeping.[52] This would suggest that if GER is causally related to SIDS/apnea, there is more GER in the prone position. However, Bhat et al have demonstrated that there is no significant difference between the amount of acid reflux and the number of obstructive apnea events in premature infants in the prone or supine position.[53] This would suggest that there are other factors independent of GER that are playing a role in SIDS associated with infant positioning. As mentioned previously, studies have shown that there is a poor correlation between GER and apnea in premature infants.[51] By bypassing the stomach, transpyloric feeds have the potential to decrease GER. Malcolm et al have demonstrated decreased apnea and bradycardia in very low birthweight premature infants who have been fed with nasal duodenal or nasojejunal feeds.[54] Malcolm et al's study implicates GER as playing a potential role in the pathogenesis of apnea and bradycardia in premature infants. The Nissen fundoplication is thought to be effective in reducing GER. Valusek et al retrospectively reviewed their experience in using fundoplication to decrease GER in 81 infants with ALTE. These patients had been resistant to medical management of GER. Only 3% of the 81 patients with ALTE had recurrent ALTE after fundoplication. Follow-up after fundoplication was 173 days.[55] The results of this study suggest that GER can be implicated as playing a role in ALTE.

Fortunately, the duration of ALTE is rare beyond 8 months of age, and the frequency of ALTE diminishes as the infant matures. However, ALTE is of concern in more vulnerable infants, such as premature infants and infants with other medical conditions. An analysis of current studies suggests that, in most infants with ALTE, GER is not the cause. MII combined with polysomnogram and pH monitoring appears to be valuable in evaluating the potential causal effect of GER in ALTE in selected infants.[7]

GERD AND FEEDING REFUSAL

Food refusal and aversion to feeding are frequently encountered in pediatric practice, occurring in about 25% of otherwise normally developing infants and 80% of those with developmental handicaps.[56,57] *Feeding refusal* and *feeding difficulty* are terms that are used mainly to describe symptoms such as refusal to eat, uncoordinated sucking and swallowing, gagging, vomiting, or excessive crying and irritability during feeds. These symptoms have been reported as being related to GERD.[58-61]

It is well documented that symptoms of GERD vary by age, and the verbal description of intensity, localization, and severity may be unreliable until at least 8 years of age in normally developed children.[62-65] For infants with crying and feeding difficulties, it is the parents who bring them to medical attention. In this population, persistent crying, irritability, back arching, feeding, and sleep difficulties have been proposed as the equivalent of heartburn in adults. However, in 2 controlled studies using proton pump inhibitors (PPIs) in distressed infants, there was an equal decrease in distressed behavior in the PPI treatment and in the placebo groups.[66,67] This suggests that there is no evidence that acid-suppressive therapy is effective in infants who present with inconsolable crying alone. In another study of infants seen in clinic for a complaint of irritability and fussiness, it was reported that they had more feeding difficulties, were less responsive to treatment, and had more maternal stress.[68] Children with GERD tend to present more frequently with food refusal, regurgitation, vomiting, and abdominal pain.[69] Older children and adolescents with GERD typically complain of heartburn or substernal burning.[9,70]

There have been several attempts to define the relationship between GERD and feeding refusal. Regurgitation, irritability, and vomiting are common in infants with physiologic GER. These symptoms are indistinguishable from regurgitation, irritability, and vomiting associated with other conditions such as food allergies or colic.[7,9,71-74] Although older case series suggest that reflux disease is a cause of infant feeding difficulty, no prospective studies have proven causation and none have demonstrated resolution of symptoms after GERD therapy.[58] In these older studies, it is also unclear if eosinophilic esophagitis was present and contributing to feeding difficulties. A recent double-blinded, placebo-controlled trial showed no improvement in feeding difficulties following lansoprazole therapy compared with placebo in infants with GERD.[67] In children 1 to 5 years of age, another study demonstrated that anorexia or feeding refusal was occasionally a symptom of erosive esophagitis.[69] In a retrospective study of pH-MII studies, only 38% of perceived pain-related symptoms (eg, back arching, crying, restlessness, thrashing, screaming, fussiness) were associated with nonacid reflux episodes. This suggests that acid reflux does not appear to play a major role in infants perceived to have pain-related symptoms.[75] Nelson et al followed 6- to 12-month-old infants with frequent regurgitation and compared them to a control group. One year later, regurgitation had stopped in all patients, but eating and meals were still considered unpleasant events. These findings suggest that infant regurgitation may result in imprinting a "negative eating experience" that persists for a longer period than the regurgitation itself.[76] Further, Duca et al report that young children with a history of vomiting after feeding (GER or other reasons) may have difficulty in accepting feeds, despite having no alteration of oral and pharyngeal phases of swallowing.[77] The proposed hypothesis to explain this is that initial acid exposure of the mucosal chemoreceptors and nerve endings in the esophagus triggers afferent signals to the spinal nerves, which are transmitted to the brain. The brain perceives the sensation as pain or discomfort. The neurochemical alterations induced in this pathway by repeated reflux episodes appear to persist even after the original noxious stimulus (eg, vomiting, GERD) resolves. This leaves the child with a hypersensitivity to any bolus movement along the esophagus, including swallowed food. Peripheral and central sensitization are believed to be important mechanisms for this ongoing heightened perception of esophageal sensation (visceral sensitivity) resulting in food refusal.[78] Further studies on this exciting theory are needed to expand our knowledge, which will hopefully lead to clinical application.

The role of impaired mother-child interactions in the perpetuation of feeding difficulties in GERD was identified by Dellert et al. They demonstrated a high level of maternal worrying and severe frustration at feeding times in families and infants with GERD.[58] More recently, Karacetin et al suggested that maternal anxiety and force feeding convert GER to GERD, which promotes maladaptive behaviors.[79] However, how much parental psychopathology contributes to feeding difficulties in GERD is not yet defined.

GERD AND INSUFFICIENT WEIGHT GAIN

Infants who present with feeding difficulties and poor weight gain are among the most vexing patients physicians may encounter, both in the primary and tertiary care setting. Poor weight gain, particularly in an infant, is a red flag that requires immediate evaluation. There are many excellent references on the evaluation of failure to thrive.[4]

Though poor weight gain may be associated with GERD, this has been demonstrated in only a minority of infants.[7,80] It has been suggested that excessive regurgitation may lead to caloric insufficiency, but there are usually other associated disorders leading to weight loss. One example is the severe reduction in feeding volumes to prevent regurgitation and vomiting, which adversely affects weight gain. Another may be abnormal sucking and swallowing, which causes decreased oral intake. There are also abnormal feeding practices by the parent/caregiver, such as "forcing" feeds irrespective of hunger cues or intrusive feeding behaviors, which may result in the development of enhanced feeding difficulties and poor intake and weight gain.[81] In conjunction with a gastroenterologist, a skilled feeding therapist can be helpful in the assessment and management of these patients.

GERD IN RESPIRATORY AND EAR, NOSE, AND THROAT DISORDERS

In adult patients with GERD, approximately one-third will have extraesophageal symptoms.[82] These include pulmonary, ENT, and dental conditions. In children under the age of 5 years, the overall prevalence of GER varies from 2% to 25%.[83] This broad range of prevalence is related to the variability of defining and diagnosing GER. The prevalence of extraesophageal symptoms in children with GERD was determined in a systematic review of the literature by Tolia and Vandenplas.[84] By pooling data from several prospective and retrospective observational studies and a few controlled studies and case series, they determined that, in more than 2000 pediatric patients with GER, 57.7% had generalized respiratory symptoms, 40.2% had dental erosions, 13.2% had concurrent asthma, 6.2% had pneumonia, 4.2% had sinusitis, and 2.1% had otitis media.

GERD AND ASTHMA

In a large retrospective database evaluation of children over the age of 2 years from a major children's hospital, El-Serag et al found the prevalence of asthma in children with GERD was doubled compared to controls (13.2% versus 6.8%, respectively; $p < 0.0001$).[85] Conversely, asthmatic patients had an average prevalence of GER of 23.4% versus 3.8% of controls, though studies varied greatly in estimating prevalence of GER in asthmatics (from 19.3% and 65%). The studies that used objective measures such as endoscopic or pH probe monitoring results tended to show higher rates when compared to studies that made the diagnosis of GER based on symptom reporting.[84,86-89] When the subset of asthmatics who do not have atopic disease is considered, the prevalence rate of GER is much higher than in atopic patients, suggesting the likelihood that in nonatopic patients, GER may be a significant factor in triggering asthma.[90-92] Despite the dramatic variability of rates described in these various studies, it is clear that there is an increased likelihood of having concurrent asthma and GERD.

The association of asthma and GERD does not provide a clear understanding of whether there is a cause and effect phenomenon or merely a coexistence of 2 diagnoses that are common in the pediatric population. What seems to be apparent is that the 2 conditions may exacerbate each other. Multiple authors cite 2 proposed hypotheses of GER inducing asthma: (1) microaspiration and (2) acidification of the esophagus triggering a vagally mediated bronchospastic reflex. Mechanisms by which asthma increases the likelihood of GER include an increased pressure gradient between the thorax and abdomen and decreased LES tone secondary to hyperinflation and asthma medication effect.[93-98]

In contrast to adults, many children with asthma may not report gastrointestinal symptoms. Therefore, studies using symptom questionnaires may underestimate rates of concurrent asthma and GER. The use of objective testing, especially pH-MII, and endoscopy will reveal a larger cohort of patients who have "silent reflux." Therefore, it is recommended to consider such testing in asthmatics who do not respond adequately to conventional asthma treatments or those who have frequent exacerbations.

Many reports have shown that combined pH-MII monitoring is superior to pH probe alone in diagnosing GERD in patients with respiratory disease.[11,15-30,99-102] Other diagnostic modalities (eg, bronchoscopy and endoscopy) can give additional specific histologic data, but these may not correlate with clinical findings. As mentioned in an earlier section of this chapter, the presence of LAM in the lungs is no longer considered to have adequate sensitivity or specificity to be reliable.[31-34,103]

In patients with refractory or persistent asthma, antireflux therapy (either medical or surgical) seems to improve asthma symptoms and reduce the need for asthma medications. However, there may be no concurrent change in pulmonary function.[104-110] Therapy with PPIs is more effective than H2 receptors antagonists.[111] Benefits from therapy with PPIs may not be evident with brief courses of treatment. Earlier studies had revealed similar efficacy with prokinetic agents (eg, cisapride), though this agent is not in current use in the United States.[112]

GERD AND COUGH

An evaluation of 72 infants and children with chronic cough by Hollinger and Sanders revealed that the most common cause was asthma (32%) with sinusitis as a close second (23%). GER was found to be causal in 15% to 27% of patients with chronic cough.[113,114] Several studies in adults have shown that MII may be the best way to determine that GER is temporally associated with chronic cough.[115-117] In a study by Borrelli et al[118] of 45 children who had concurrent cough and GER, 79% did not have typical GER symptoms. MII evaluation of these children revealed that in patients with cough-related reflux, there was an increase in weakly acidic GER and alkaline GER. This suggests that while a positive response to antireflux therapy may be considered diagnostic,[119] in a subset of patients with chronic reflux, cough may not improve with acid-suppressive therapy alone. In addition, in Borrelli et al's report, only patients with erosive esophagitis, who were used as controls, showed an increase in esophageal acid exposure time and delay in esophageal clearance of acid, suggesting that the reflux index calculated on MII is not reliable in patients with reflux-related cough.[118] The pathophysiology of GER-associated cough is similar to that of asthma with neurally mediated reflexes and micro- or macroaspiration triggering reflex cough.[120] Bronchial hypersensitivity induced by GER may be a third mechanism.[121] The nature of the cough (ie, wet-moist [likely sinusitis] versus dry [asthma]) may help guide therapy.[119,122] An empiric course of therapy with PPIs, H2 receptor antagonists, and/or prokinetics for 8 to 12 weeks may be warranted prior to performing extensive testing.[123]

GERD AND EAR, NOSE, AND THROAT DISORDERS

A variety of otolaryngologic entities, (eg, rhinopharyngitis, sinusitis, laryngitis, globus pharyngeus, vocal cord granuloma, stridor, laryngomalacia, and subglottic stenosis) may be associated with GER. Laryngopharyngeal reflux of gastric juices seem to be the postulated pathogenetic mechanism. A study of 14 children with rhinopharyngitis who underwent nasopharyngeal pH monitoring by Concentin and Narcy revealed an increased incidence of acidic pH in the rhinopharyngitis group compared to controls.[124] Yellon et al's group performed distal esophageal biopsies on 101 children undergoing a variety of ENT procedures and found statistically significant associations of esophagitis in patients with asthma (75%; p < 0.006), cough (81%; p < 0.001), apnea (75%; p < 0.001), sinusitis (100%;

p < 0.001), laryngomalacia (21%, p = 0.006), posterior glottic erythema (83%, p < 0.001), and posterior glottic edema (81%, p = 0.002). A somewhat less significant association was seen in patients with recurrent croup (p = 0.04), stridor (p = 0.04), and subglottic stenosis (p = 0.02).[125] In a case report by Putnam and Orenstein of a child with hoarseness and GER (diagnosed by pH probe and esophageal biopsy), resolution of symptoms with treatment of GER was demonstrated.[126]

El-Serag et al's large database review also noted an association between GER and sinusitis, though interestingly it showed that otitis media occurred less frequently in children with GER compared to those without GER.[85] Tasker et al and Abd El-Fattah et al showed that assay of pepsin and pepsinogen in middle ear fluid in patients with otitis media with effusion was highly suggestive of GER-induced otitis media.[127,128] He et al described similar findings though in less frequent rates of association.[129] Rozmanic's group performed dual pH monitoring on 27 children with chronic ENT disorders and found that 55.6% had pathologic GER suggesting no significant association between GER and ear disorders.[130] They recommend using this modality in patients with refractory ENT disorders to determine if GER may be contributing to chronic symptoms. This study corroborates the finding of Bouchard et al who performed a retrospective analysis of patients with ENT disorders who underwent pH probe analysis. Their findings suggested slightly increased GER in patients with sinusitis, stridor, laryngitis, and laryngomalacia, and no correlation in patients with otitis.[131] In summary, the association of ENT disorders with GER in children is still questionable though in refractory patients, especially with sinusitis and laryngitis, this association should be considered. Based on these studies, dual pH monitoring and esophageal histology are more definitive diagnostic modalities. Empiric antireflux therapy in ENT conditions is not recommended.

CONCLUSION

GERD in the pediatric population is a common entity. Review of the literature suggests that there are many extraesophageal manifestations of GER, including apnea, ALTE, feeding problems, poor weight gain, asthma, cough, and ENT disorders. Our analysis of the current literature suggests the following:

- Apnea/ALTE/SIDS is not causally related to GER except in selected cases, which may include preterm infants.

- In children with feeding difficulty, the literature supports a temporal association with GER. Unfortunately, medical therapy for GER does not resolve the feeding issues, suggesting a more complex neurobehavioral component may exist. These issues will require further study.

- In children with insufficient weight gain (failure to thrive), there has been little evidence that GER is solely responsible. There is a complex interaction between social, behavioral, and physical factors that plays a role as well.

- In children with asthma, chronic cough, and chronic sinusitis that are refractory to conventional therapy, silent GER must be considered. Following a brief empiric trial of a PPI, combined pH-MII and esophageal biopsy is recommended in elucidating this potential relationship in the individual patient.

- While some patients with a variety of other ENT disorders may also have GER, the causal relationship between these disorders is not clear. Empiric therapy for GER is not recommended in this patient population. However, objective testing for GER maybe warranted in selected patients who are unresponsive to conventional therapy.

While there is currently a tremendous interest in a causal relationship between GER and these various conditions in pediatric patients, the data linking these conditions directly to GER are tenuous. This may be partially due to the variety of diagnostic modalities used in previous trials. With the advent of pH-MII, more targeted data can be obtained. Prospective, randomized, controlled trials with adequate sample sizes are needed to adequately determine the true prevalence, long-term complications and response to treatment, of GER in patients with presumed EES.

REFERENCES

1. Jadcheria SR. Gastroesophageal reflux in the neonate. *Clin Perinatol.* 2002;29:135-158.
2. Gold BD. Gastroesophageal reflux disease: could intervention in childhood reduce the risk of later complications? *Am J Med.* 2004;117(suppl 5A):23S-29S.
3. Kawahara H, Dent J, Davidson G. Mechanisms responsible for gastroesophageal reflux in children. *Gastroenterology.* 1997;113(2):399-408.
4. Vandenplas Y. Gastroesophageal reflux. In: Wyllie R, Hyams JS, ed. *Pediatric Gastroenterology and Liver Disease.* 4th ed. Philadelphia, PA: Elsevier; 2011:232.
5. Vandenplas Y, Hassall E. Mechanisms of gastroesophageal reflux and gastroesophageal reflux disease. *J Pediatr Gastroenrerol Nutr.* 2002;35:119-136.
6. Chawla S, Seth D, Mahajan P, Kamat D. Gastroesophageal reflux disorder: a review for primary care providers. *Clin Pediatr.* 2006;45:7-13.
7. Vandenplas Y, Rudolph CD, Di Lorenzo C, et al. Pediatric gastroesophageal reflux practice guidelines: joint recommendations of the North American Society for Pediatric Gastroenterology, Hepatology and Nutrition (NASPGHAN) and the European Society for Pediatric Gastroenterology Hepatology and Nutrition (ESPGHAN). *J Pediatr Gastroenterol Nutr.* 2009;49:498-547.
8. Michail S. Gastroesophageal reflux. *Pediatr Rev.* 2007;28:101-110.
9. Nelson SP, Chen EH, Syniar GM, Christoffel KK. Prevalence of symptoms of gastroesophageal reflux during infancy: a pediatric practice based survey, Pediatric Practice Research Group. *Arch Pediatr Adolesc Med.* 2000;154:569-572.
10. Cucchiara S, Campanozzi A, Greco L, et al. Predictive value of esophageal manometry and gastro-esophageal pH monitoring for responsiveness of reflux disease to medical therapy. *Am J Gastroenterol.* 1996;91(4):680-685.
11. Heine RG, Cameron DJ, Chow CW, Hill DJ, Catto-Smith AG. Esophagitis in distressed infants: poor diagnostic agreement between esophageal pH monitoring and histopathologic findings. *J Pediatr.* 2002;140:14-19.
12. Gilger MA, Gold BD. Pediatric endoscopy: new information from the PEDS-CORI project. *Current Gastroenterol Rep.* 2005;7:234-239.
13. Croffie JM, Fitzgerald JF, Molleston JP, et al. Accuracy and tolerability of the Bravo catheter-free pH capsule in patients between the ages of 4 and 18 years. *J Pediatr Gastroenterol Nutr.* 2007;45:559-563.
14. Hochman JA, Favaloro-Sabatier J. Tolerance and reliability of wireless pH monitoring in children. *J Pediatr Gastroenreol Nutr.* 2005;41:411-415.
15. Sondheimer JM. Continuous monitoring of distal esophageal pH: a diagnostic test for gastroesophageal reflux in infants. *J Pediatr.* 1980;96(5):804-807.
16. Johnson CF, DeMeester TR. Development of the 24 hour pH monitoring composite scoring system. *J Clin Gastroenterol.* 1986;(suppl 1):52-58.
17. Vandenplas Y, Goyvaerts H, Helven R, Sacre L. Gastroesophageal reflux as measured by 24 hour pH monitoring in 509 healthy infants screened for risk of SIDS. *Pediatrics.* 1991;88(4):834-840.
18. Vandenplas Y, Sacré-Smits L. Continuous 24 hour pH monitoring in 285 infants 0-15 months old. *J Pediatr Gastroenterol Nutr.* 1987;6:220-224.
19. Cucchiara S, Staiano A, Gobio Casali L, Boccieri A, Paone FM. Value of the 24 hour intraesophageal pH monitoring in children. *Gut.* 1990;31:129-133.
20. Wenzl TG, Moroder C, Trachterna M, et al. Esophageal pH monitoring and pH measurement: a comparison of two diagnostic tests for gastroesophageal reflux. *J Pediatr Gastroenterol Nutr.* 2002;34:519-523.
21. Wenzl TG. Evaluation of gastroesophageal reflux events using multichannel intraluminal electrical impedance. *Am J Med.* 2003;115(suppl 3A):161S-165S.
22. Loots CM, Benninga MA, Davidson GP, Omari TI. Addition of multichannel intraluminal impedance to standard pH monitoring increases the yield of symptom associated analysis in infants and children with gastroesophageal reflux. *J Pediatr.* 2009;154:248-252.

23. López-Alonso M, Moya MJ, Cabo JA, et al. Twenty-four hour esophageal impedance pH monitoring in healthy preterm neonates: rate and characteristics of acid, weakly acidic and weakly alkaline gastroesophageal reflux. *Pediatrics.* 2006;118:e299-e308.

24. Francavilla R, Magistà AM, Bucci N, et al. Comparison of esophageal pH and multiple intraluminal impedance testing in pediatric patients with suspected gastroesophageal reflux. *J Pediatr Gastroenterol Nutr.* 2010;50(2):154-160.

25. Salvatore S, Arrigo S, Luini C, Vandenplas Y. Esophageal impedance in children: symptom-based results. *J Pediatr.* 2010;157:949-954.

26. Mousa HM, Rosen R, Woodley FW, et al. Esophageal impedance monitoring for gastroesophageal reflux. *J Pediatr Gastroenterol Nutr.* 2011;52(2):129-139.

27. Pilic D, Fröhlich T, Nöh F, et al. Detection of gastroesophageal reflux in children using combined multichannel impedance and pH measurement: data from the German Pediatric Impedance Group. *J Pediatr.* 2011;158:650-654.

28. Rosen R, Hart K, Nurko S. Does reflux monitoring and multichannel intraluminal impedance change clinical decision making? *J Pediatr Gastroenterol Nutr.* 2011;52(4):404-407.

29. Salvatore S, Hauser B, Devreker T, et al. Esophageal impedance and esophagitis in children: any correlation? *J Pediatr Gastroenterol Nutr.* 2009;49(5):566-570.

30. Loots CM, van Wijk MP, Blondeau K, et al. Interobserver and intraobserver variability in pH impedance analysis between 10 experts and automated analysis. *J Pediatr.* 2012;160(3):444-446.

31. Nussbaum E, Maggi JC, Mathis R, Galant SP. Association of lipid laden macrophages and gastroesophageal reflux in children. *J Pediatr.* 1987;110(2):190-194.

32. Rosen R, Fritz J, Nurko A, Simon D, Nurko S. Lipid-laden macrophage index is not an indication of gastroesophageal reflux related respiratory disease in children. *Pediatrics.* 2008;121(4):e879-e884.

33. Farrell S, McMaster C, Gibson D, Shields MD, McCallion WA. Pepsin in bronchiolar lavage fluid: a specific and sensitive method of diagnosing gastroesophageal reflux related pulmonary aspiration. *J Pediatr Surg.* 2006;41:289-293.

34. Starosta V, Kitz R, Hartl D, Marcos V, Reinhardt D, Griese M. Bronchoalveolar pepsin, bile acids, oxidation and inflammation in children with gastroesophageal reflux disease. *Chest.* 2007;132(5):1557-1564.

35. He Z, O'Reilly RC, Mehta D. Gastric pepsin in middle ear fluid of children with otitis media: clinical implications. *Current Allergy Asthma Rep.* 2008;8(6):513-518.

36. Abd El-Fattah AM, Abdul Maksoud GA, Ramadan AS, Abdalla AF, Abdel Aziz MM. Pepsin assay: a marker for reflux in pediatric glue ear. *Otolaryngol Head Neck Surg.* 2007;136(3):464-470.

37. Oren J, Kelly D, Shannon DC. Identification of a high risk group for sudden infant death syndrome among infants who were resuscitated for sleep apnea. *Pediatrics.* 1986;77:495-499.

38. National Institutes of Health Consensus Development Conference on Infantile Apnea and Home Monitoring, Sept 29 to Oct 1, 1986. *Pediatrics.* 1987;79:292-299.

39. Vandenplas Y, Hauser B. Gastroesophageal reflux, sleep patterns, apparent life threatening event and sudden infant death. The point of view of a gastroenterologist. *J Pediatr.* 2000;159:726-729.

40. Veereman-Wauters G, Bochner A, Van Caillie-Bertrand M. Gastroesophageal reflux in infants with a history of near miss sudden infant death. *J Pediatr Gastroenterol Nutr.* 1991;12:319-323.

41. Herbst JJ, Minton SD, Book LS. Gastroesophageal reflux causing respiratory distress and apnea in newborn infants. *J Pediatr.* 1979;95(5):763-768.

42. Herbst JJ, Book LS, Bray PF. Gastroesophageal reflux in the "near miss" sudden infant death syndrome. *J Pediatr.* 1978;92(1):73-75.

43. Menon AP, Schefft GL, Thach BT. Apnea associated with regurgitation in infants. *J Pediatr.* 1985;106(4):625-629.

44. Newman LJ, Russe J, Glassman MS, et al. Patterns of gastroesophageal reflux (GER) in patients with apparent life-threatening events. *J Pediatr Gastroenterol Nutr.* 1989;8(2):157-160.

45. Kahn A, Rebuffat E, Sottiaux M, Dufour D, Cadranel S, Reiterer F. Lack of temporal relation between acid and reflux in the proximal esophagus and cardiorespiratory events in sleeping infants. *Eur J Pediatr.* 1992;151(3):208-212.

46. Paton JY, Macfadyen U, Williams A, Simpson H. Gastroesophageal reflux and apneic pauses during sleep in infancy-no direct relation. *Eur J Pediatr.* 1990;149(10):680-686.

47. Walsh JK, Farrell MK, Keenan WJ, Lucas M, Kramer M. Gastroesophageal reflux in infants: relation to apnea. *J Pediatr.* 1981;99(2):197-201.

48. Wenzl TG, Schenke S, Peschgens T, Silny J, Heimann G, Skopnik H. Association of apnea and nonacid gastroesophageal reflux in infants: investigations with the intraluminal impedance technique. *Pediatr Pulm.* 2001;31:144-149.

49. Mousa H, Woodley FW, Metheney M, Hayes J. Testing the association between gastroesophageal reflux and apnea in infants. *J Pediatr Gastroenterol Nutr.* 2005;41:169-177.

50. Magistà AM, Indrio F, Baldassarre M, et al. Multichannel intraluminal impedance to detect relationships between gastroesophageal reflux and apnea of prematurity. *Dig Liver Dis.* 2007;39(3):216-221.

51. Peter CS, Sprodowski N, Bohnhorst B, Silny J, Poets CF. Gastroesophageal reflux and apnea of prematurity: no temporal relationship. *Pediatrics.* 2002;109(8):8-11.

52. Skadberg BT, Morild I, Markestad T. Abandoning prone sleeping: effect on the risk of sudden infant death syndrome. *J Pediatr.* 1998;132(2):340-343.

53. Bhat RY, Rafferty GF, Hannam S, Greenough A. Acid gastroesophageal reflux in convalescent preterm infants: effect of posture and relationship to apnea. *Pediatr Res.* 2007;62(8):620-623.

54. Malcolm WF, Smith PB, Mears S, Goldberg RN, Cotten CM. Transpyloric tube feeding in very low birthweight infants with suspected gastroesophageal reflux: impact on apnea and bradycardia. *J Perinatol.* 2009;29(5):372-375.

55. Valusek PA, St Peter SD, Tsao K, Spilde TL, Ostlie DJ, Holcomb GW 3rd. The use of fundoplication for prevention of apparent life threatening events. *J Pediatr Surg.* 2007;42:1022-1024.

56. Reilly SM, Skuse DH, Wolke D, Stevenson J. Oral motor dysfunction of children who fail to thrive: organic or non-organic? *Dev Med Child Neurol.* 1999;41:115-122.

57. Chatoor I, Ganiban J. Food refusal by infants and young children: diagnosis and treatment. *Cogn Behav Pract.* 2003;10:138-146.

58. Dellert SF, Hyams JS, Treem WR, Geertsma MA. Feeding resistance and gastroesophageal reflux in infancy. *J Pediatr Gastroenterol Nutr.* 1993;17:66-71.

59. Mathisen B, Worrall L, Masel J, Wall C, Shepherd RW. Feeding problems in infants with gastroesophageal reflux disease: a controlled study. *J Paediatr Child Heath.* 1999;35:163-169.

60. Hyman PE. Gastroesophageal reflux: one reason why baby won't eat. *J Pediatr.* 1994;125(6 pt 2):S103-S109.

61. Catto-Smith AG, Machida H, Butzner JD, Gall DG, Scott RB. The role of gastroesophageal reflux in paediatric dysphagia. *J Pediatr Gastroenterol Nutr.* 1991;12:159-165.

62. von Baeyer CL, Spagrud LJ. Systematic review of observational (behavioral) measures of pain for children and adolescents age 3-28 years. *Pain.* 2007;127:140-150.

63. Stanford EA, Chambers CT, Craig KD. The role of developmental factors in predicting young children's use of a self support scale for pain. *Pain.* 2006;120:16-23.

64. Beyer JE, McGrath PJ, Berde CB. Discordance between self report and behavioral pain measures in children aged 3-7 years after surgery. *J Pain Symptom Manage.* 1990;350-356.

65. Shields BJ, Palermo TM, Powers JD, Grewe SD, Smith GA. Predictors of a child's ability to use a visual analogue scale. *Child Care Health Dev.* 2003;29:281-290.

66. Moore DJ, Tao BS, Lines DR, Hirte C, Heddle ML, Davidson GP. Double blind placebo controlled trial of omeprazole in irritable infants with gastroesophageal reflux. *J Pediatr.* 2003;143:219-223.

67. Orenstein SR, Hassall E, Furmaga-Jablonska W, Atkinson S, Raanan M. Multicenter, double blind, randomized, placebo controlled trial assessing the efficacy and safety of proton pump inhibitor lansoprazole in infants with symptoms of gastroesophageal reflux disease. *J Pediatr.* 2009;154:514-520.

68. Miller-Loncar C, Bigsby R, High P, Wallach M, Lester B. Infant colic and feeding difficulties. *Arch Dis Child.* 2004;89(10): 908-912.

69. Gupta SK, Hassall E, Chiu YL, Amer F, Heyman MB. Presenting symptoms of nonerosive and erosive esophagitis in pediatric patients. *Dig Dis Sci.* 2005;51(5):858-863.

70. Ashorn M, Ruuska T, Karikoski R, Laippala P. The natural course of gastroesophageal reflux disease in children. *Scan J Gastroenterol.* 2002;37(6):638-641.

71. Salvatore S, Vandenplas Y. Gastroesophageal reflux and cow milk allergy: is there a link? *Pediatrics.* 2002;110:972-984.

72. Hill DJ, Heine RG, Cameron DJ, et al. Role of food protein intolerance in infants with persistent distress attributed to reflux esophagitis. *J Pediatr.* 2000;136:641-647.

73. Vandenplas Y, Koletzko S, Isolauri E, et al. Guidelines for the diagnosis and management of cow's milk protein allergy in infants. *Arch Dis Child.* 2007;92:902-908.

74. Barr RG. Colic and crying syndromes in infants. *Pediatrics.* 1998;102(5 suppl E):1282-1286.

75. Garza JM, Kaul A. Gastroesophageal reflux, eosinophilic esophagitis, and foreign body. *Pediatr Clin N Am.* 2010;57:1331-1345.

76. Nelson SP, Chen EH, Syniar GM, Christoffel KK. One year follow up of symptoms of gastroesophageal reflux during infancy. Pediatric Practice Research Group. *Pediatrics.* 1998;102(6):E67.

77. Duca AP, Dantas RO, Rodrigues AA, Sawamura R. Evaluation of swallowing in children with vomiting after feeding. *Dysphagia.* 2008;23(2):177-182.

78. Anand P, Aziz Q, Willert R, van Oudenhove L. Peripheral and central mechanisms of visceral sensitization in man. *Neurogastroenterol Motil.* 2007;19(suppl1):29-46.

79. Karacetin G, Demir T, Erkan T, Cokugras FC, Sonmez BA. Maternal psychopathology and psychomotor development of children with GERD. *J Pediatr Gastroenterol Nutr.* 2011;53(4):380-385.

80. Vandenplas Y, Hauser B, Devreker T, Mahler T, Degreef E, Veereman-Wauters G. Gastroesophageal reflux in children: symptoms, diagnosis, and treatment. *J Pediatr Sciences.* 2011;3(4):2-20.

81. Levy Y, Levy A, Zangen T, et al. Diagnostic clues for identification of nonorganic versus. Organic causes of food refusal and poor feeding. *J Pediatr Gastroenterol Nutr.* 2009;48:355-362.

82. Jaspersen D, Kulig M, Labenz J, et al. Prevalence of extra-oesophageal manifestations in gastro-oesophageal reflux disease: an analysis based on the ProGERD Study. *Aliment Pharmacol Ther.* 2003;17:1515-1520.

83. Nelson SP, Chen EH, Syniar GM, Christoffel KK. Prevalence of symptoms of gastroesophageal reflux during childhood: a pediatric practice-based survey. Pediatric Practice Research Group. *Arch Pediatr Adolesc Med.* 2000;154:150-154.

84. Tolia V, Vandenplas Y. Systematic review: the extra-oesophageal symptoms of gastro-oesophageal reflux disease in children. *Aliment Pharmcol Ther.* 2009;29:258-272.

85. El-Serag HB, Gilger M, Kuebeler M, Rabeneck L. Extraesophageal associations of gastroesophageal reflux disease in children without neurologic defects. *Gastroenterology.* 2001;121:1294-1299.

86. Størdal K, Johannesdottir GB, Bentsen BS, Carlsen KC, Sandvik L. Asthma and overweight are associated with symptoms of gastro-oesophageal reflux. *Acta Paediatr.* 2006:95:1197-1201.

87. Debley JS, Carter ER, Redding GJ. Prevalence and impact of gastro-esophageal reflux in adolescents with asthma: a population based study. *Pediatr Pulmonol.* 2006;41:475-481.

88. Barakat M, Sherit AH, El-Kady ZM, Hasanean MH. Patterns of gastrointestinal symptoms in children with a wheezy chest. *Gut.* 2006;55(suppl 5):G-403.

89. Chopra K, Matta SK, Madan N, Iyer S. Association of gastroesophageal reflux (GER) with bronchial asthma. *Indian Pediatr.* 1995;32:1083-1086.

90. Yüksel H, Yilmaz O, Kirmaz C, Aydogdu S, Kasirga E. Frequency of gastroesophageal reflux disease in nonatopic children with asthma-like airway disease. *Resp Med.* 2006;100:393-398.

91. Khoshoo V, Haydel R. Effect of antireflux treatment on asthma exacerbations in nonatopic children. *J Pediatr Gastroenterol Nutr.* 2007;44:331-335.

92. Dal Negro RW, Turco P, Micheletto C, et al. Cost analysis of GER-induced asthma: a controlled study versus. Atopic asthma of comparable severity. *Resp Med.* 2007;101:1814-1820.

93. Hughes DM, Spier S, Rivlin J, Levison H. Gastroesophageal reflux during sleep in asthmatic patients. *J Pediatr.* 1983;102:666-672.

94. Harding SM. Recent clinical investigations examining the association of asthma and gastroesophageal reflux. *Am J Med.* 2003;115(suppl 3A):39S-44S.

95. Goldenhersh MJ, Ament M. Asthma and gastroesophageal reflux in infants and children. *Immunol Allergy Clin North Am.* 2001;21(3):439-448.

96. Alexander JA, Hunt LW, Patel AM. Prevalence, pathophysiology, and treatment of patients with asthma and Gastroesophageal reflux disease. *Mayo Clin Proc.* 2000;75:1055-1063.

97. Turbyville JC. Applying principles of physics to the airway to help explain the relationship between asthma and gastroesophageal reflux. *Med Hypotheses.* 2010;74(6):1075-1080.

98. icciardolo FL, Gaston B, Hunt J. Acid stress in the pathology of asthma. *J Allergy Clin Immunol.* 2004;113:610-619.

99. Harding SM, Guzzo MR, Richter JE. 24-h esophageal pH testing in asthmatics: respiratory symptom correlation with esophageal acid events. *Chest.* 1999;115:654-659.

100. Condino AA, Sondheimer J, Pan Z, Gralla J, Perry D, O'Connor JA. Evaluation of gastroesophageal reflux in pediatric patients with asthma using impedance-pH monitoring. *J Pediatr.* 2006;149:216-219.

101. Rosen R, Nurko S. The importance of multichannel intraluminal impedance in the evaluation of children with persistent respiratory symptoms. *Am J Gastroenterol.* 2004;99:2452-2458.

102. Wenzl TG, Silny J, Schenke S, Peschgens T, Heimann G, Skopnik H. Gastroesophageal reflux and respiratory phenomenon in infant: status of the intraluminal impedance technique. *J Pediatr Gastroenterol Nutr.* 1999;28(4):423-428.

103. Krishnan U, Mitchell JD, Tobias V, Day AS, Bohane TD. Fat laden macrophages in tracheal aspirates as a marker of reflux aspiration: a negative report. *J Pediatr Gastroenterol Nutr.* 2002;35:309-313.

104. Field SK, Sutherland LR. Does medical anti-reflux therapy improve asthma in asthmatics with gastroesophageal reflux? A critical review of the literature. *Chest.* 1998;114:275-283.

105. Writing Committee for the American Lung Association Asthma Clinical Research Centers; Holbrook JT, Wise RA, Gold BD, et al. Lansoprazole for children with poorly controlled asthma. *JAMA.* 2012;307(4):373-381.

106. Klaus A, Swain JM, Hinder RA. Laparoscopic antireflux surgery for supraesophageal complications of gastroesophageal reflux disease. *Am J Med.* 2001;111(suppl 8A):202S-206S.

107. Hassal E. Decisions in diagnosing and managing chronic gastroesophageal reflux disease in children. *J Pediatr.* 2005;146(3 suppl):S3-S12.

108. Katz PO, Castell DO. Medical therapy of supraesophageal gastroesophageal reflux disease. *Am J Med.* 2000;108(suppl 4A):170S-177S.

109. Pitcher DE, Pitcher WD, Martin DT, Curet MJ. Antireflux surgery does not reliably correct reflux related asthma. *Gastrointest Endosc.* 1996;43(4):433.

110. Sontag SJ, O'Connell S, Khandelwal S, et al. Asthmatics with gastroesophageal reflux: long term results of a randomized trial of medical and surgical antireflux therapies. *Am J Gastroenterol.* 2003;98:987-999.

111. Tolia V, Ferry G, Gunasekaran T, Huang B, Keith R, Book L. Efficacy of lansoprazole in the treatment of gastroesophageal reflux disease in children. *J Pediatr Gastroenterol Nutr.* 2002;35:S308-S318.

112. Vandenplas Y; ESPGHAN Cisapride Panel. European Society for Pediatric Gastroenterology, Hepatology and Nutrition. Current pediatric indications for cisapride. *J Pediatr Gastroenterol Nutr.* 2000;31:480-489.

113. Hollinger LD, Sanders AD. Chronic cough in infants and children: an update. *Laryngoscope.* 1991:101:596-605.

114. Khoshoo V, Edell D, Mohnot S, Haydel R Jr, Saturno E, Kobernick A. Associated factors in children with chronic cough. *Chest.* 2009;136:811-815.

115. Irwin RS, Madison JM. Diagnosis and treatment of chronic cough due to gastro-esophageal disease and post nasal drip. *Pulm Pharmcol Ther.* 2002;15:261-266.

116. Blondeau K, Dupont LJ, Mertens V, Tack J, Sifrim D. Improved diagnosis of gastro-esophageal reflux in patients with unexplained chronic cough. *Aliment Pharmacol Ther.* 2007;25:723-732.

117. Sifrim D, Dupont L, Blondeau K, Zhang X, Tack J, Janssens J. Weakly acidic reflux in patients with chronic unexplained cough during 24 hour pressure, pH and impedance monitoring. *Gut.* 2005;54:449-454.

118. Borrelli O, Marabotto C, Mancini V, et al. Role of gastroesophageal reflux in children with unexplained chronic cough. *J Pediatr Gastroenterol Nutr.* 2011;53(3):287-292.

119. Goldsobel AB, Chipps BE. Cough in the pediatric population. *J Peds.* 2010;156(3):352-358.

120. Ing AJ, Ngu MC, Breslin AB. Pathogenesis of chronic persistent cough associated with gastro-esophageal reflux. *Am J Respir Crit Care Med.* 1994;149:160-167.

121. Pauwels A, Blondeau K, Dupont L, Sifrim D. Cough and gastroesophageal reflux: from the gastroenterologist end. *Pulm Pharmacol Ther.* 2009;22:135-138.

122. Chang AB. Cough. *Pediatr Clin N Am.* 2009;56:19-31.

123. Rudolph CD, Mazur LJ, Liptak GS, et al; North American Society for Pediatric Gastroenterology and Nutrition. Guidelines for evaluation and treatment of gastroesophageal reflux in infants and children: recommendations of the North American Society for Pediatric Gastroenterology and Nutrition. *J Pediatr Gastroenterol Nutr.* 2001;(32 suppl):S1-S3.

124. Concentin P, Narcy P. Nasopharyngeal pH monitoring in infants and children with chronic rhinopharyngitis. *Int J Pediatr Otorhinolaryngol.* 1991;22:249-256.

125. Yellon RF, Coticchia J, Dixit S. Esophageal biopsy for the diagnosis of gastroesophageal reflux-associated otolaryngologic problems in children. *Am J Med.* 2000;108(suppl 4A):131S-138S.

126. Putnam PE, Orenstein SR. Hoarseness in a child with gastroesophageal reflux. *Acta Pediatr.* 1992;81:635-636.

127. Tasker A, Dettmar PW, Panetti M, Koufman JA, P Birchall J, Pearson JP. Is gastric reflux a cause of otitis media with effusion in children? *Laryngoscope.* 2002;112(11):1930-1934.

128. Abd El-Fattah AM, Abdul Maksoud GA, Ramadan AS, Abdalla AF, Abdel Aziz MM. Pepsin assay: a marker for reflux in pediatric glue ear. *Otolaryngol Head Neck Surg.* 2007;136:464-470.

129. He Z, O'Reilly RC, Bolling L, et al. Detection of gastric pepsin in middle ear fluid of children with otitisi media. *Otolaryngol Head Neck Surg.* 2007;137:59-64.

130. Rozmanic V, Velepic M, Ahel V, Bonifacic D, Velepic M. Prolonged esophageal pH monitoring in the evaluation of gastroesophageal reflux in children with chronic tubotympanal disorders. *J Pediatr Gastroenterol Nutr.* 2002;34:278-280.

131. Bouchard S, Lallier M, Yazbeck S, Bensoussan A. The otolaryngologic manifestations of gastroesophageal reflux: when is a pH study indicated? *J Pediatr Surg.* 1999;34(7):1053-1056.

Financial Disclosures

Dr. Sheeja K. Abraham has no financial or proprietary interest in the materials presented herein.

Dr. Lisa S. Cassani has no financial or proprietary interest in the materials presented herein.

Dr. Donald O. Castell is a consultant and speaker for Sandhill Scientific, a consultant for Torax Medical, and a speaker for Takeda.

Dr. John O. Clarke has no financial or proprietary interest in the materials presented herein.

Dr. Sidney Cohen has no financial or proprietary interest in the materials presented herein.

Dr. Anthony J. DiMarino Jr has no financial or proprietary interest in the materials presented herein.

Dr. Joan S. Di Palma has no financial or proprietary interest in the materials presented herein.

Dr. Dina Halegoua-DeMarzio has no financial or proprietary interest in the materials presented herein.

Dr. Susan M. Harding has no financial or proprietary interest in the materials presented herein.

Dr. Christine Herdman has no financial or proprietary interest in the materials presented herein.

Dr. David A. Katzka has no financial or proprietary interest in the materials presented herein.

Dr. Britta Magnuson has no financial or proprietary interest in the materials presented herein.

Dr. Vikneswaran Namasivayam has no financial or proprietary interest in the materials presented herein.

Dr. Athena Papas has no financial or proprietary interest in the materials presented herein.

Dr. Rebecca O. Ramirez has no financial or proprietary interest in the materials presented herein.

Dr. Lindsey B. Roenigk has no financial or proprietary interest in the materials presented herein.

Dr. Mabi Singh has no financial or proprietary interest in the materials presented herein.

Dr. Joseph R. Spiegel has a royalty agreement with KayPentax, Inc regarding a patent on a portable endoscopy system.

Dr. Michael F. Vaezi receives research funds from Takeda Pharmaceuticals.

Index

acid reflux. *See also* esophageal reflux; extraesophageal reflux; gastric acids; gastroesophageal reflux disease (GERD); laryngopharyngeal reflux (LPR); nasopharyngeal reflux; nocturnal GERD
    asthma and, 11–12
    control of, 92
    cough preceding, 11
    mechanisms of, 2, 3–5
    in sleep arousal, 77–78
acid-suppressive therapy
    for extraesophageal reflux, 60, 72
    for GERD-related cough, 62
        in children, 104
    postnasal drip and, 65
adolescents, presenting GERD symptoms in, 98
airflow obstruction, 37
airway
    neuroinflammatory mediators in, 35
    protective reflexes of, 57
albuterol, 37
alcohol use, laryngeal cancer and, 65–66
allergies, postnasal drip and, 64–65
amorphous calcium phosphate toothpaste, 92
antireflux barrier, 3
antireflux surgery, impedance monitoring after, 27. *See also* fundoplication
anxiety, 8
apnea, sleep
    obstructive, 13
    in pediatric population, 98, 100–101

apparent life-threatening events (ALTE), in pediatric population, 98, 100–101
aspiration, GER-related, 8–9. *See also* microaspiration
    in chronic obstructive pulmonary disease, 44
    in cystic fibrosis, 44
    diagnosis of, 43
    in lung transplant recipients, 45
    pathophysiology of, 43
    in pulmonary fibrosis and systemic sclerosis, 44
    treatment of, 43
asthma, GERD-related, 8, 11–12, 36
    in chronic cough, 40, 61
    controversies of, 39–40
    diagnosis and treatment of, 37
    epidemiology of, 37
    National Asthma Education and Prevention Program treatment guidelines for, 37
    in pediatric population, 103–104
    response to GER treatment in, 38–39
    triggers of, 36

barium esophagram
    for chronic cough, 40
    in pediatric population, 98–99
Barrett's esophagus, 6, 55
benzodiazepine, in nocturnal GERD, 79
bile acids, 6, 43–45, 57
bitter taste, 86

bronchitis, eosinophilic, 40
bronchoalveolar lavage fluid, 43, 45
bronchoconstriction, 11, 35, 37

cancer, laryngeal, 8, 53–54, 55, 65–66, 68, 72
central sensitization, 7–8
chemosensory changes, 87
chest pain, noncardiac, 8
children. *See* pediatric population
choking, in laryngopharyngeal reflux, 52, 100
chronic obstructive pulmonary disease, 44
cigarette smoking
        in chronic laryngitis, 63
        in laryngeal cancer, 53, 65–66
cough
        chronic, 8, 10–11, 42–43, 72
                causes of, 40, 61
                controversies of, 42
                defined, 40
                GER treatment outcomes in, 41–42
                in pediatric population, 104
                pH monitoring in, 61–62
                testing and diagnosis of, 40–41
                treatment of, 41, 62
        postinfectious, 40
        reflux as trigger in, 10, 55
cystic fibrosis, 44

dental caries, 88
dental erosion, 8, 9, 85, 88–89, 93
        diagnosis of, 89–91
        management of, 91–92
        salivary hypofunction and, 86
diaphragmatic crural fibers, 3
diaphragmatic hernia, 98
duodenogastroesophageal reflux, 6
dysphagia, in laryngopharyngeal reflux, 52

ear, middle
        chronic inflammation of, 72
        extraesophageal reflux in, 54
endoscopy, 22
        in pediatric population, 99
        transnasal fiber optic, 52
esomeprazole, 80
esophageal-bronchial reflux, 10
esophageal peristalsis, intact, 5
esophageal reflux
        in sleep arousal, 81
        sleep disturbance and, 75–81
esophageal syndromes, 1–2
esophagitis, 6
        classification of, 22–23
esophagus
        acid clearance in, 5
                during sleep, 12
        atresia of, 98
        biopsy of in children, 99
        bronchoconstriction and acid reflux in, 35
        injury to
                gastric refluxate in, 7
                mucosal defense against, 7–8

interactions with lungs, 42
        mucosal erythema of, 85
        peristaltic actions of, 57
        pH monitoring in, 42–43
        physiology of, 35–36
        sensitization of, 7–8
extraesophageal reflux, 1–2, 86–89
        in chronic rhinosinusitis, 54
        in otitis media, 54
        in pediatric population, 97–106

feeding refusal/difficulties, 101–102
fluoride, in tooth remineralization, 92
fundoplication
        after lung transplantation, 45
        asthma outcomes with, 38–39
        for chronic GER-related cough, 41
        for extraesophageal reflux, 60
        for GER-related aspiration, 44
        impedance monitoring after, 27
        reducing laryngeal symptoms, 55

gastric acids, 6–7
        in chronic cough, 40
        in extraesophageal reflux, 57
        secreted during sleep, 12
        in tracheobronchial tree and lungs, 43
gastric refluxate, 6
gastroesophageal junction
        competence of, 3
        protective structures of, 57
gastroesophageal reflux disease (GERD). *See also* laryngopharyngeal reflux (LPR); nasopharyngeal reflux; nocturnal GERD
        definition of, 1–2
        diagnostic algorithm for, 29
        esophageal acid clearance and, 5
        in esophageal injury, 6–7
        evaluation of, 21, 29
                ambulatory pH monitoring, 22–25
                endoscopic, 22
                impedance testing, 25–27
                nonacid reflux in, 28
        extraesophageal manifestations of
                definition of, 1–2
                pathophysiology of, 2–14
        management algorithm for, 30
        Montreal definition of, 2
        perception of, 7–8
gastroschisis, 98
globus, 51–52, 104
gum recession, 90–91

halitosis, 85, 87
heartburn, 8
        nocturnal, 12–13, 78
        sinusitis and, 64
Helicobacter pylori, in sinusitis, 64
hiatal hernia, 2, 3, 4, 98
hoarseness, reflux-associated, 52, 63–64, 105
hypnotics, in nocturnal GERD, 79

impedance monitoring, 99
   advantages of, 25–27
   for chronic cough, 61–62
   disadvantages of, 27
   for extraesophageal reflux, 60, 61
   for hoarseness, 64
   for laryngopharyngeal reflux, 72
   for nocturnal GERD, 79
   in pediatric population, 98
infants
   feeding difficulties in, 101–102
   insufficient weight gain in, 102–103
   presenting GERD symptoms in, 98
intra-abdominal/intrathoracic pressure, increased, 11, 61

laryngeal cancer, 8, 53–54, 55, 65–66, 68, 72
laryngitis, reflux-induced, 8, 9–10, 51–53
   causes of, 62
   controversies of, 72
   signs and symptoms of, 62–63
laryngomalacia, 104
laryngopharyngeal reflux (LPR), 51
   causes of, 72
   in children, 104–105
   chronic laryngitis in, 51–53
   chronic rhinosinusitis in, 54
   controversies of, 55, 72
   diagnostic tools for, 58–59
   evident for GERD association with, 68
   gastroenterologist's perspective on, 57–69
   laryngeal cancer in, 53–54
   otitis media in, 54
   otolaryngologist's perspective on, 51–55
   pH monitoring in, 59–60
   potential signs of, 58
   subglottic stenosis in, 54
   surgical therapy for, 69
   symptoms of, 57
   treatment algorithm for, 68
   treatment recommendations for, 72
laryngoscopy, 72
   for chronic laryngitis, 52, 53
   for laryngopharyngeal reflux, 58
   for reflux-induced laryngitis, 9
larynx
   abnormal, 59
   cancer of, 65–66
   erythema and edema of, 62–63
   inflammation of, 62–63
   irritation and inflammation of, 51
   normal tissue of, 58
   ulceration of, 58, 62
Los Angeles classification, modified, 22–23
lower esophageal sphincter (LES), 3
   hypertension of, 2, 3, 4
   transient relaxation of (TRLES), 3–4
      in asthma, 11–12
      bronchoconstriction and, 35
      in pediatric population, 97–98
lung transplant recipients, GER-related aspiration in, 45

lungs
   fibrosis of, 12, 44
   gastric acid secretions in, 43
   interactions with esophagus, 42
   physiology of, 35–36
microaspiration, 11, 12
   bronchoconstrictive response to, 35
   in extraesophageal reflux, 57
mouth sores, 85, 87

nasopharyngeal reflux, 54
   in sinusitis, 64
nocturnal GERD, 75
   clinical importance of, 79
   complications of, 79
   pathophysiology of, 76–79
   prevalence of, 75–76
   in sleep arousal, 77–78
   as sleep arousal trigger, 81
   treatment of, 80
nonacid reflux
   in chronic cough, 42
   role of, 28
nonerosive reflux disease (NERD), 6, 7
   conditions associated with, 8
nuclear scintigraphy, in pediatric population, 98

obesity, 4–5
omeprazole, 62–63
omphalocele, 98
oral manifestations, 85–93
oral mucosa
   erythema of, 87
   irritation of, 87
   ulcerations of, 87
otitis media, 54, 65, 105
otolaryngologic manifestations, 51–55, 61–69
   in children, 104–105

paradoxical vocal fold dysfunction, 66–67
paranasal sinuses, chronic inflammation of, 54, 55, 72
pediatric population
   apnea and apparent life-threatening events in, 100–101
   asthma in, 103–104
   cough in, 104
   diagnosis in, 98–99
   ENT disorders in, 104–105
   extraesophageal manifestations in, 97–106
   feeding refusal in, 101–102
   insufficient weight gain in, 102–103
   respiratory and ENT disorders in, 103
pepsin
   in esophageal injury, 6–7
   in extraesophageal reflux, 57
   laryngeal exposure to, 55
   in middle ear, 54
   in nasopharynx, 54
peripheral sensitization, 7
pH-elevating oral sprays, 92

pH monitoring. *See also* impedance monitoring
    ambulatory, 22–25
        advantages of, 23–24
        disadvantages of, 24–25
    for asthma, 37
    in children, 98, 99
        with asthma, 104
        with feeding difficulties, 102
        with GERD, 105
    for chronic cough, 41, 42–43, 61–62
    for hoarseness, 64
    for laryngopharyngeal reflux, 59–60, 61, 72
    for nocturnal GERD, 77, 79
    for reflux-induced laryngitis, 9–10
    for sinusitis, 64
polysomnography, for nocturnal GERD, 77
postnasal drip, 40, 61, 64–65
proton pump inhibitor (PPI) therapy, 7, 60, 65
    asthma outcomes with, 38, 39–40, 104
    for chronic cough, 11, 42, 62
    for chronic laryngitis, 52, 63
    dental erosions and, 9
    in distressed infants, 101
    in GERD diagnosis, 29–30
    for hoarseness, 63–64
    for laryngopharyngeal reflux, 67, 68, 72
    for postnasal drip, 65
    for sleep disturbance, 80
    for subglottic stenosis, 67
proud restoration, 89–90
psychological stress, 8
ptyalism, 87
pulmonary disease, GERD-induced
    aspiration, 43–45
    asthma, 36–40
    chronic cough, 40–43
    future directions in, 45
    pathophysiological mechanisms of, 35–36
pulmonary fibrosis, 12, 44

radionucleotide scanning, 43
reflux symptom index, 65
regurgitation
    GERD and, 102
    sinusitis and, 64
respiratory disorders, pediatric, 103
rhinopharyngitis, 104
rhinosinusitis, chronic, 54

saliva
    in acid neutralization, 57
    drooling of, 87
    impaired production of, 5
    increasing flow of, 92
    protective role of, 85–86
    during sleep, 76
salivary hypofunction, 86
Savary-Miller classification, modified, 23

sialorrhea, 87
silent nocturnal reflux group, 78
sinusitis, 64, 72
    in children, 105
    postnasal drip and, 64–65
Sjögren's syndrome, salivary hypofunction and, 86
sleep
    reflux during, 12–13, 76–77
    swallowing during, 76–77.97–98
sleep disturbance, GERD-related, 81
    clinical importance of, 79
    pathophysiology of, 76–79
    prevalence of, 75–76
    treatment of, 80
Sleep Heart Health Study, nocturnal reflux predictors of, 76
sour taste, 86
spatiation, 8
steroids, in GERD, 37
subglottic stenosis, 54, 67
surgical therapy, asthma outcomes with, 38–39
swallowing, during sleep, 76–77, 97–98
systemic sclerosis, GER-related aspiration in, 44

taste disturbances, 87
theophylline, 11, 37
tonsillar pillars, irritation of, 88
tooth. *See also* dental caries; dental erosion
    remineralization of, 92
    restoration of, 92
    surface loss in, 88–89
        diagnosing, 89–92
tracheal intubation, 67
tracheal stenosis, 54
tracheobronchial tree, gastric acid secretions in, 43
transient receptor potential channels (TRPV1), 7

upper airway cough syndrome, 40
upper GI series, in children, 98–99
uvula, irritation of, 88

vagal neuropathy, 55
vagal reflex arc stimulation, 57
visceral hypersensitivity, 7
vocal cords
    granuloma of in children, 104
    postviral dysfunction of, 66–67

water brash, 85, 87
weight gain, insufficient, 102–103

xerophthalmia, 86
xerostomia, 5, 86, 87

zolpidem, in nocturnal GERD, 79